Street Mental Health Handbook

Simon Hatcher • Liz Frye • Kim Van Herk

Street Mental Health Handbook

Care Delivery Across the Spectrum of Homelessness

Springer

Simon Hatcher
University of Ottawa and Ottawa
Inner City Health
Ottawa, ON, Canada

Liz Frye
Street Medicine Institute
Pittsburgh, PA, USA

Kim Van Herk
Ottawa Inner City Health
Ottawa, ON, Canada

ISBN 978-3-032-00662-2 ISBN 978-3-032-00663-9 (eBook)
https://doi.org/10.1007/978-3-032-00663-9

This Springer imprint is published by the registered company Springer Nature Switzerland AG
The registered company address is: Gewerbestrasse 11, 6330 Cham, Switzerland

Preface

The fact that we felt compelled to write a book on street mental health is not something to be celebrated—it is a reflection of systemic failure. Over the past decade, homelessness has grown at an alarming rate in many parts of the world. This surge is not merely a consequence of individual misfortune, but rather a result of cumulative breakdowns in housing systems, mental health services, addiction treatment frameworks, and economic policies. The increase in visible homelessness mirrors deeper structural inequities and a persistent inability of social systems to respond effectively to those most in need.

With the rise in homelessness has come a growing movement of street medicine—health care delivered directly to individuals who live on the streets, in encampments, or within emergency shelters. Within this evolving field, the provision of mental health care has become increasingly prominent. Yet while physical health services are relatively well-integrated into street medicine models, mental health care remains underdeveloped, fragmented, and often poorly resourced. There is a pressing need for guidance, reflection, and solidarity among those who choose to work in this space.

We wrote this book to address that need. Our primary audience is the front-line clinicians—physicians, nurses, outreach workers, social workers, and others—who are new to the field of street mental health or are seeking to deepen their understanding of it. For those already embedded in this work, we hope it will serve as a practical and reflective guide that acknowledges the unique challenges and rewards of working with people who are homeless and living with mental illness.

This is not a policy manual, nor is it a treatment guideline. Readers will not find a policy discussion about safer supply, protocols for managing treatment-resistant depression, or step-by-step instructions for conducting trauma-focused therapy. Such resources already exist and are valuable in their own right. Rather, this book aims to ground the work of street mental health within the lived realities of the people it serves. We emphasize the importance of trauma—not only individual trauma, but also collective, historical, and structural trauma—and how it shapes the experience of homelessness and engagement with mental health care.

We also focus on context. The setting in which care is provided—whether a sidewalk, a tent, a shelter bed, or a drop-in center—matters. These environments form a distinct culture and community, one that is often ignored or misunderstood by mainstream systems. Street mental health requires a distinct approach that is flexible, relational, and attuned to this context. The work demands humility, creativity, and a willingness to meet people where they are—literally and figuratively.

This book is also a reflection of our shared experiences. Between us, we have several decades of working in street-based mental health services across North America. Simon Hatcher is a psychiatrist who has worked with Ottawa Inner City Health in Canada for the past 10 years. Liz Frye is a psychiatrist who has provided street-based psychiatric care in the United States since 2008 and currently serves as Chair of the Board of Directors of the Street Medicine Institute. Kim Van Herk is an advanced practice psychiatric nurse who has worked with Ottawa Inner City Health since 2008. What unites us is a belief in the dignity and humanity of people experiencing homelessness and a commitment to reducing suffering through meaningful clinical engagement.

We do not claim to have all the answers. Much of what is important in this field has not yet been formally researched or codified. Many insights have been gained through trial, error, and the wisdom of those we serve. Our goal is to share what we have learned in a way that is honest, grounded, and helpful. Ultimately, we hope this book contributes to a larger conversation about how mental health care can be reimagined and delivered in ways that are just, inclusive, and responsive to the needs of society's most marginalized members.

Ottawa, ON, Canada — Simon Hatcher
Pittsburgh, PA, USA — Liz Frye
Ottawa, ON, Canada — Kim Van Herk

Acknowledgments

We would first like to acknowledge all the people we have met on the streets—individuals whose resilience, honesty, and lived experiences have profoundly shaped our understanding of suffering, survival, and human dignity. Their stories have been our most powerful teachers, offering lessons that no textbook or classroom could provide.

Simon Hatcher would also like to express his deep gratitude to the wise and skilled nurses and other health workers who have guided and inspired him throughout his work. Their professionalism, insight, and unwavering dedication have been a constant source of learning. More than anything, they have shown him the critical importance of compassion—not as a vague ideal, but as a daily practice rooted in humility, patience, and courage.

This gratitude extends especially to Amanda Ahmed, Stephanie Muron, and Thenu Kirupamoorthy, whose clinical acumen and empathy have shaped the ethos of his work. Most of all, Simon wishes to thank Kim, who not only manages him with remarkable skill and tact but also serves as the moral compass of the Inner City Team. Her integrity, wisdom, and steady leadership help hold everything together, often in the most difficult of circumstances.

And lastly to Julie, whose love and comradeship keeps me honest.

Liz Frye would like to thank Emma Lo and Katie Koh, whose thoughtful and nuanced perspectives have helped her sort through complex clinical challenges; Andie Silva, an up-and-coming street medicine rock star, for sharing her expertise; and Tony Carino, for opening her eyes to what a robust street psychiatry program can accomplish. Liz is indebted to Sophie Roe, without whom her chapters may never have seen the light of day, for her editing eye and willingness to help out in a pinch.

Liz feels profound gratitude for the friendship, love, and encouragement of Jim Withers, Corinne Feldman, Pat Perri, Brett Feldman, Joel Hunt, Kevin Sullivan, and Kaitlin Schwan. Their commitment to social justice, indefatigable fight against structurally violent systems, and passion for street medicine inspire Liz every day.

Liz would also like to thank her husband, Kevin, for always holding down the fort and reminding her to eat and take breaks. Words are wholly insufficient to express her gratitude for his unwavering love, support, and encouragement to pursue her dreams.

Kim would like to express her deep gratitude to the Inner City team and clients, from the past, present, and future, who she has had the privilege to grow up with. Thank you for your patience with my scattered brain, my horrible technology skills, and for liking my loud laugh. You have such a deep place in my heart; we have seen each other through so much, and your hugs and our shared laughs have kept me going. Simon, you are a trusted friend in this work and that makes it fun, makes me learn, and keeps me on my toes. Thank you for all the opportunities you have shared with me along the way.

Kim would like to thank Josh, Sophia, and Annika for being the very best.

Nomenclature

Homeless as a noun as in “the homeless” but this solely defines a person by the absence of a home. Better to use homeless as an adjective

People who are “vulnerably housed”—academics like it but it is clumsy

“Street involved”—not necessarily homeless

The Canadian Observatory on Homelessness describes four types of living situations: (i) unsheltered, living on the streets, (ii) emergency sheltered, those staying on homeless shelters, (iii) provisionally accommodated whose accommodation is temporary, and (iv) at risk of homelessness which refers to people whose situation is precarious or does not meet public health and safety standards. In practice, people frequently move between these situations (Gaetz et al. 2012).

The UN has defined homelessness as “a condition where a person or household lacks habitable space with security of tenure, rights and ability to enjoy social relations, including safety; and includes the following categories of people as those experiencing homelessness: people living on the streets or other open spaces; people living in temporary or crisis accommodation; people living in severely inadequate and insecure accommodation, such as slums or informal settlements; and people who lack access to affordable housing” (UN 2020, p. 2).

Contents

Trauma

1

The most useful way to understand what is going on and how to help in a population of people who are homeless is through a trauma-informed lens. That is why we are starting this book with an introduction to trauma and how to take it into account when encountering individuals who are vulnerably housed.

1.1 What Is Trauma?

Trauma is defined in the Oxford English Dictionary as "*A psychic injury, esp. one caused by emotional shock the memory of which is repressed and remains unhealed.*" It was first used in 1894 by the psychologist and philosopher William James, "*Certain reminiscences of the shock fall into the subliminal consciousness, where they can only be discovered in 'hypnoid' states. If left there, they act as permanent 'psychic traumata', thorns in the spirit, so to speak*" (James, 1894). These definitions include the *event*, the *experience* of an individual "the shock," and the *effect* on the exposed person "the psychic injury," which remains "buried within the psyche." The event, the experience, and the effects are all components of trauma [1].

The event In DSM-5, the event that may cause trauma is defined as "*exposure to death, threatened death, actual or threatened serious injury or actual or threatened sexual violence*" [2]. The focus is on occasions when someone thinks they are going to die or be seriously hurt. The DSM-5 definition then goes on to state that trauma may be by "*direct exposure, witnessing the trauma, learning that the trauma happened to a close relative or friend or indirect exposure to aversive details of the trauma usually in the course of professional duties.*"

In the International Classification of Diseases-11 [3] the trauma event is defined as "*Exposure to an event or situation (either short- or long-lasting) of an extremely threatening or horrific nature. Such events include, but are not limited to, directly experiencing natural or human-made disasters, combat, serious accidents, torture, sexual violence, terrorism, assault or acute life-threatening illness (e.g., a heart attack); witnessing the threatened or actual injury or death of others in a sudden,*

S. Hatcher et al., *Street Mental Health Handbook*,
https://doi.org/10.1007/978-3-032-00663-9_1

unexpected, or violent manner; and learning about the sudden, unexpected or violent death of a loved one." The extension of indirect exposure to trauma so that the person affected doesn't have to witness or experience the trauma is controversial. Also, neither definition includes neglect which can have serious long-term consequences.

The experience As well as the potentially traumatic event are the emotional, psychological, and physiological responses an individual experiences *after* encountering a distressing or life-threatening event. An event that may be traumatizing for one person may not be for another.

The effect When an event overwhelms a person's ability to cope, this may result in long-term effects that can shape how they perceive and interact with the world. This may for example include changes in how people view the world, resulting in hypervigilance and increased arousal, or difficulty controlling their emotions in stressful situations.

Who develops consequences after being exposed to trauma is very dependent on the individual, what may seem overwhelming to one person may not be for someone else. Important factors that affect the development of post-traumatic stress disorder include genetic predisposition; previous trauma exposure; the severity and duration of the trauma especially if it involves interpersonal violence; and the presence or absence of strong social support.

An important distinction to make here is that all traumas involve loss but not all losses involve trauma. So, for example, the expected death of a loved one is a loss but not necessarily a traumatic event as defined in both DSM-5 or ICD-11.

1.2 How Common Is the Experience of Trauma in People Who Are Homeless?

The experience of trauma is common among people experiencing homelessness. Studies consistently show that individuals who are homeless have a significantly higher rate of trauma exposure compared to the general population. Trauma can be both a cause and a consequence of homelessness, and many people experiencing homelessness have histories of childhood adversity, abuse, or violence.

Adverse childhood events (ACEs) are defined as abuse (physical, emotional, and sexual), neglect (physical and emotional), and household challenges (mental illness in adults, intimate partner violence, parental separation, incarceration of adults, and substance abuse in adults) experienced before the age of 18. A screening questionnaire, ACEs Aware, is a ten-item questionnaire that produces an ACE score that can be used to screen populations (https://www.acesaware.org/). Studies in the late 1990s beginning at Kaiser Permanente found clear associations between the number of ACEs and leading causes of death including heart disease, asthma, cancer, diabetes as well as depression and substance abuse [4]. A systematic review from 2021 [5] of nearly 17,000 homeless individuals from 29 studies found a lifetime prevalence of one or more adverse childhood experiences (ACE's) in 89% of homeless adults and a lifetime prevalence of four or more ACEs of 54%. The same group conducted an analysis of mental health outcomes in 2235 homeless individuals in Canada, revealing a mean Adverse Childhood Experiences (ACE) score of 4.4 [6]. The study found that 58.6% of participants had experienced 4 or more ACEs, while 28.1% had experienced 7 or more. These figures are strikingly higher than those reported in the original ACE study of housed participants, where only 12% experienced 4 or more ACEs and 0.9% experienced 7 or more. This represents an almost fivefold increase for 4 or more ACEs and a 32-fold increase for 7 or more ACEs in the homeless population compared to the housed population. Among the ACEs reported, household criminal justice involvement was the least common (30.4%), while emotional abuse was the most prevalent (62.0%). Notably, 38% of participants reported experiencing sexual abuse. The study also revealed significant gender differences, with women generally reporting a higher prevalence of ACEs. However, this gender disparity did not extend to parental separation, substance abuse, or criminal justice system involvement in the household. These findings underscore the disproportionate burden of adverse childhood experiences among homeless individuals and highlight the potential long-term impact of early-life trauma on housing stability and mental health outcomes.

1.3 Trauma as a Risk Factor for Homelessness

A systematic review of factors that predicted becoming homeless found that adverse life events in childhood including sexual, physical, and emotional abuse, family problems, and foster care were all strong predictors of becoming homeless [7]. A history of childhood trauma also predicted poorer outcomes in people who received Housing First [8]. In adulthood, fleeing abuse is a common pathway into homelessness with this being cited as a reason for homelessness in 20% of women and 5% of men [9].

1.4 Trauma as a Consequence of Homelessness

Trauma is not just a historical event but living precariously continually exposes people to trauma and dangerous situations including assault, robbery, and sexual violence and lack of security. A systematic review of street crime victimization amongst homeless adults found that compared to the general population, assault occurred 11 times more frequently, robbery 12 times more often, and theft 20 times as frequently [10]. A 2023 study of 851 women who were homeless and using substances in Arizona [11] found that three-quarters of them had experienced sexual assault and abuse during their lifetime and nearly a quarter had experienced this in the last 30 days. Also, nearly all the women had experienced significant loss, including forced displacement and separation from children. In people who present to hospital with physical trauma, those who are homeless are more likely to experience an assault or self-inflicted injury and less likely to experience an unintentional injury compared to those who are housed [12]. Also people who are homeless are three times more likely to present to emergency departments with intentional self-injury than individuals who are housed [13].

1.5 The Effects of Trauma

The experience of trauma alters brain circuits responsible for emotion regulation, executive function, threat detection, contextual processing, and fear learning [14]. In individuals with post-traumatic stress disorder (PTSD) or similar conditions, these physiological changes persist even after the traumatic event has passed. The amygdala plays a central role in these brain circuits, with its function modulated by other cortical and subcortical structures, including the hippocampus, insula, and prefrontal areas. During recovery from PTSD, brain changes occur primarily within the areas involved in the fear response, such as the amygdala and hippocampus, with evidence suggesting increased connectivity between these regions and the prefrontal cortex [15]. This often involves a normalization of previously heightened activity in the amygdala and a strengthening of the prefrontal cortex's ability to inhibit fear responses.

Trauma leaves a lasting imprint on both the body and mind, creating a "template" through which future experiences are processed. This template can be reactivated by seemingly minor stressors, which may appear inconsequential to outside observers. Consequently, trauma survivors become "primed" to respond to situations and relationships that share emotional characteristics with past traumatic events or evoke a perceived threat. This heightened sensitivity can show itself in various ways affecting daily functioning and interpersonal relationships.

Early experience of trauma, often from people who are supposed to care for them such as family, results in individuals learning that those who care for them can hurt them. Due to early life experiences, the roles of carer and abuser can blend together.

Trauma that involves violation of trust is particularly common in people who are homeless. One study reported this as occurring in 40% of a sample of 77 adults who were chronically homeless [16] . However paradoxically people with a history of betrayal of trust were more likely to seek out patient care [17]. This means that trust, especially trust in health care professionals who are trying to care, is a major issue. A nurse or doctor approaching someone who has been abused may cause feelings of fear and reenactment of the original trauma. Also racialized and/or marginalized populations may have had previous negative encounters with health care providers and the health care system. For example, some of our Inuit homeless clients have had particularly negative reactions towards getting TB tests done because they have literally experienced family members be locked away in TB sanitoriums for months. As much as health care providers are well-meaning, sometimes we knowingly or unknowingly are part of people's trauma stories and experiences with the health care system.

Trauma is often remembered but always reenacted. What this means is that people who have experienced trauma, especially early in life, repeatedly relive the trauma in the present. For example, women who experience childhood sexual or physical abuse will often have repeated relationships with abusive men as adults [18]. The reasons for reenactments can vary and may be adaptive or maladaptive [19]. Some victims of trauma need to put into actions that which can't be put into words, so people express their inner world through what they do rather than speaking about what is happening. Often when this happens clinicians feel awkward or that they are somehow in the role of an abuser without quite knowing how they got there. Reenactments can also be a way of trying to achieve mastery of a past trauma "this time I'll get it right." Alternatively, the defenses that people use to avoid reexperiencing trauma have the opposite effect and can create situations they were trying to avoid. For example, avoiding abandonment can lead to dependency on clinicians, which is often pathologized and can lead to rejection by the clinician or services which were trying to help them.

Another way of thinking about reenactment is through attachment theory. Attachment theory described by [20] explains how individuals manage their relationship with carers during times of stress, such as separation from those carers. The description of different attachment styles can vary but all distinguish between secure and insecure attachment styles. Insecure attachment styles can be divided into anxious styles (enmeshed or fearful) and avoidant (angry-dismissive or withdrawn). The experience of repeated trauma in early life can lead to an insecure attachment style characterized by a lack of trust and a lack of a secure base. In people who are homeless, this is often seen in individuals who are labelled as "hard to engage" or "care resistant" who are excluded from services or shelter because of their disruptive behavior. A systematic review of attachment in the homeless found that in the eight studies assessed nearly two-thirds had an insecure attachment type [21]. This also affects how frontline staff relate to homeless individuals. Individuals with attachment styles characterized by high anxiety (enmeshed or fearful) made staff feel compassion and that they were able to help. However, the ambivalence and dependence of this attachment style also risked staff feeling exhausted. Alternatively, attachments styles characterized by avoidance (withdrawal or angry-dismissive) lead to feelings of frustration and low job satisfaction in staff [22]. There is also some evidence that individuals experiencing homelessness with avoidant attachment styles are less likely to improve with psychotherapy compared to other attachment styles [23]. Effective responses to insecure attachment styles usually involve elements of trauma informed care at the individual or organizational level (for example, Psychologically Informed Environments).

1.6 "Trauma Brain," the Defense Cascade, and the Window of Tolerance

Evidence from both animal and human studies show that the way the body reacts to threat follows a clearly defined path [24]. This is the "defense cascade" (sometimes also referred to as the "fear network"), Fig. 1.1, which progresses from initial freezing and orientation to flight or fight, followed by immobility (tonic immobility—frozen in fright") and finally to a fainting response ("playing dead"). Progression to

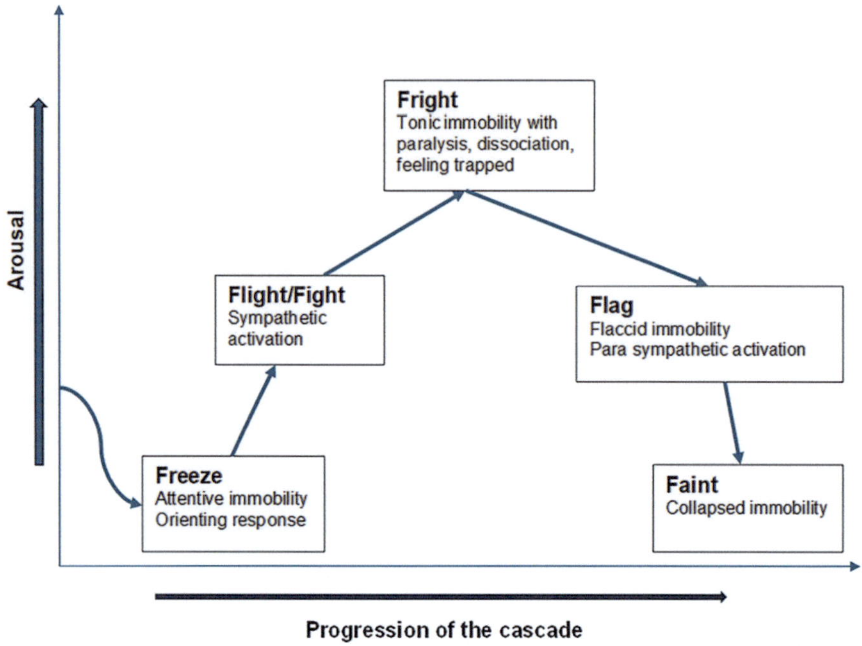

Fig. 1.1 The defense cascade

fright involves activation of the sympathetic nervous system with tachycardia, hypertension, high emotional arousal, and dissociation. Moving from fright to faint involves a protective "shut down" mediated by the parasympathetic system with a drop in arousal, slowing heart rate, low blood pressure, emotional numbing, and immobility.

The reason it is important for clinicians to know about the defense cascade is that this can become "hard wired" into the physiology of people who have been subject to repeated trauma so that any perceived threat will trigger all or part of this response. This leads to heightened vigilance and anxiety and a phenomenon referred to as a restricted "window of tolerance"where the "stress thermostat" is set too high or low and is easily triggered [25]. The window of tolerance represents the optimal zone between hyper-arousal and hypo-arousal, within which individuals typically function without strong feelings overwhelming them, Fig. 1.2. For those who have endured childhood abuse or other chronic trauma, intimate interpersonal interactions, for example with clinicians or others who say they want to help, can trigger a state of hyperarousal, as past intimate relationships have been characterized by terror, anxiety, and fear. Consequently, when forming new relationships, trauma survivors may avoid novelty, gravitating instead towards familiar patterns, even if these are ultimately destructive. The experience of trauma tends to lower the threshold for being emotionally overwhelmed, effectively narrowing the individual's window of tolerance. This concept proves valuable in informing treatment strategies aimed at supporting individuals to stay within their tolerance window.

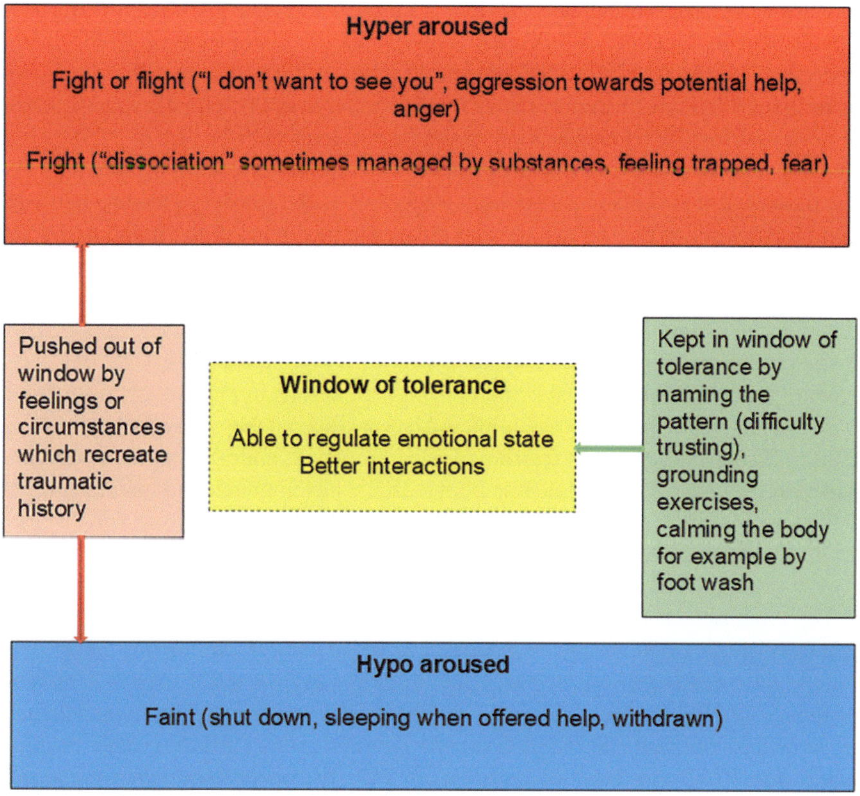

Fig. 1.2 Window of tolerance

Understanding the impact trauma has on development can help to understand behaviors, thoughts, and feelings as an adaptation to trauma rather than necessarily as sign of mental illness. For example, substance use can be seen as a way of coping with the anxiety and hypervigilance resulting from repeated trauma; creating "drama" can be seen as a learnt way of connecting when other methods have failed rather than "attention seeking" or when words have failed, for example when "no" is ignored when abuse continues.

1.7 Post-traumatic Stress Disorder, Complex Post-traumatic Stress Disorder, and Borderline Personality Disorder

Post-traumatic stress disorder (PTSD) is a diagnostic category in ICD 11 and DSM V and is defined by exposure either directly or indirectly to actual or threatened death, serious injury, or sexual violence and the presence of intrusive symptoms relating to the event; avoidance of reminders of the event; negative thoughts and mood associated with the event (the last is not a criteria in ICD11); and marked alterations in arousal that last for over a month and cause significant distress or impairment in function. A systematic review of the prevalence of PTSD in the homeless found that about 28% of people who are homeless met the diagnostic criteria for PTSD in 19 studies with a total population of 20,364 participants across seven countries [26]. However, there are some problems with the idea of PTSD. First, the diagnosis does not take into account the developmental level of the person when the trauma occurs. This is particularly important as the impact of trauma can vary significantly depending on the age and developmental level of the individual when the traumatic event occurred. For instance, trauma experienced in early childhood may have different manifestations and long-term consequences compared to trauma experienced in adulthood. Second, there is little attention given to the somatic manifestations of trauma exposure. Trauma can have significant effects on the body, leading to a range of physical symptoms and alterations in physiological functioning. Drawing from the Adverse Childhood Event research these may include chronic pain, gastrointestinal issues, cardiovascular problems, and alterations in immune function. Last, the role of attachment style in the development and maintenance of PTSD symptoms is not explicitly addressed in the current diagnostic framework - "who was there for you" after the trauma is not a consideration.

Complex Post-Traumatic Stress Disorder (cPTSD) is a diagnostic category in ICD 11 but not DSM V. It is defined as "*a disorder that may develop following exposure to an event or series of events of an extremely threatening or horrific nature, most commonly prolonged or repetitive events from which escape is difficult or impossible (for example torture, slavery, genocide campaigns, prolonged domestic violence, repeated childhood sexual or physical abuse). All diagnostic requirements for PTSD are met. In addition, cPTSD is characterized by severe and persistent (1) problems in affect regulation; (2) beliefs about oneself as diminished, defeated or worthless, accompanied by feelings of shame, guilt or failure related to the traumatic event; and (3) difficulties in sustaining relationships and in feeling close to others. These symptoms cause significant impairment in personal, family, social, educational, occupational or other important areas of functioning.*"

One Australian study of the prevalence of PTSD and complex PTSD in 206 people who were homeless found 60% with complex PTSD and 16% with PTSD, although there was some overlap with high levels of affect dysregulation, negative self-concept, and disturbances in relationships in both groups [27]. However, this does demonstrate the usefulness of the diagnosis of complex PTSD as a diagnosis in this population. A later study from Ireland of 56 homeless adults found a third with a diagnosis of complex PTSD and only 3.6% with PTSD [28]. The most prevalent interpersonal trauma was neglect. This is important, as while childhood neglect is included as an adverse childhood event, it does not meet the DSM V criteria as a traumatic event as it doesn't involve exposure to threatened death, serious injury, or sexual assault. However, "nothing matters" and is important to consider neglect as another form of trauma in this population.

One response to complex PTSD is that it is borderline personality disorder plus PTSD. Borderline personality disorder is a controversial diagnosis based on an outdated categorical understanding of personality. The diagnostic criteria include difficulty regulating emotions, unstable relationships, impulsivity, and a morbid fear of abandonment. However, these criteria are vague, subjective, and overlap with normal feelings, behaviors, and thoughts that occur in stressful situations. Despite the diagnostic criteria for borderline personality disorder stating that they are pervasive and long–standing, 25% of people diagnosed with borderline personality disorder no longer meet the criteria after 2 years and 85% at 10 years [29]. Other criticisms of the diagnosis include that it is often used in a pejorative way and to deny people access to services. It also doesn't generate many useful ideas for help and is similar to saying that someone has blue eyes—it is just a feature of who they are. Therapy for borderline personality disorder is usually limited to dialectical behavior therapy (DBT) which is rarely readily available. Also, current guidelines only recommend the use of DBT in women with borderline personality disorder with recurrent self-harm [30] which is a minority of the homeless population. Other differences between cPTSD and borderline personality disorder is that exposure to trauma is a part of the definition of cPTSD but is not necessary for the personality disorder; in cPTSD, relationships often feature avoidance, disconnection, and reenactment of trauma, while in borderline personality disorder there is often volatility with the aim of avoiding being abandoned; and cPTSD is marked by a very negative script about one self rather than the unstable self-image seen in borderline personality disorder.

1.8 Intergenerational and Institutional Trauma

Intergenerational trauma occurs when the effects of trauma are passed from one generation to the next. How this occurs is open to some debate. There is a limited evidence base in rats of change in gene expression caused by trauma that could be inherited [31]. However, what is probably more relevant are the social and policy pathways that increase the likelihood of traumatic events occurring and removing protective factors from one generation to the next. An example of this is the colonial policies to assimilate indigenous peoples in Canada. These policies remove land and cultural resources, which increase poverty, discourage traditional parenting, and provide few resources to cope with adversity. It is no surprise that data from the Canadian National Shelter Study in 2021 [32] that the proportion of shelter users who identified as indigenous was 39% compared to about 5% identifying as indigenous in the general population.

References

1. SAMHSA. SAMHSA'S concept of trauma and guidance for a trauma-informed approach. In 2014. p. 9.
2. American Psychiatric Association. Diagnostic and statistical manual of mental disorders (DSM-5). 5th ed. Washington, DC: American Psychiatric Association Publishing; 2013.
3. World Health Organization. World Health Organization. 2021 [cited 2025 Feb 12]. International Classification of Diseases, Eleventh Revision (ICD-11). Available from: https://icd.who.int/browse11

4. Felitti VJ, Anda RF, Nordenberg D, Williamson DF, Spitz AM, Edwards V, et al. Relationship of childhood abuse and household dysfunction to many of the leading causes of death in adults: the adverse childhood experiences (ACE) study. Am J Prev Med. 1998;14:245.
5. Liu M, Luong L, Lachaud J, Edafati H, Reeves A, Hwang SW. Adverse childhood experiences and related outcomes among adults experiencing homelessness: a systematic review and meta-analysis. Lancet Public Health. 2021;6(11):E836–47.
6. Liu M, Mejia-Lancheros C, Lachaud J, Latimer E, Aubry T, Somers J, et al. Overall and Gender-specific Associations between Dimensions of Adverse Childhood Experiences and Mental Health Outcomes among Homeless Adults: Associations Générales et Sexospécifiques Entre les Dimensions des Expériences Défavorables de L'enfance et les. Canadian J Psychiatry [Internet]. 2021:070674372198915. Available from: http://journals.sagepub.com/doi/10.1177/0706743721989158
7. Nilsson SF, Nordentoft M, Hjorthøj C. Individual-level predictors for becoming homeless and exiting homelessness: a systematic review and meta-analysis. J Urban Health [Internet]. 2019;96(5):741–50. Available from: https://link.springer.com/article/10.1007/s11524-019-00377-x
8. Mejia-Lancheros C, Lachaud J, Aubry T, Wiens K, O'Campo P, Stergiopoulos V, et al. Multi-trajectory group profiles of well-being and associated predictors among adults experiencing homelessness and mental illness: findings from the At Home/Chez Soi study. Toronto site Soc Psychiatry Psychiatr Epidemiol. 2022;57(1):67–81.
9. Homelessness: How does it happen? – Statistics Canada [Internet]. [cited 2025 May 6]. Available from: https://www.statcan.gc.ca/o1/en/plus/5170-homelessness-how-does-it-happen
10. Ellsworth JT. Street crime victimization among homeless adults: a review of the literature. Vict Offender. 2019;14(1):96–118.
11. Greene A, Korchmaros JD, Frank F. Trauma experience among women who have substance use disorders and are homeless or near homeless. Community Ment Health J [Internet]. 2023;60(2):233–43. Available from: https://link.springer.com/article/10.1007/s10597-023-01162-6#citeas
12. Kovacs MS, Cucher DJ, Thiessen N, Ghaemmaghami V, Watt JM, Hu CK. Outcomes and characteristics differ between homeless and housed trauma patients following the COVID-19 pandemic. Injury [Internet] 2025 Jan 1 [cited 2025 Jan 12];56(1). Available from: https://pubmed.ncbi.nlm.nih.gov/39632167/
13. Giannouchos T, Mehmood G, Yue D. Suicide and self-injury-related emergency department visits and homelessness among adults 25-64 years old from 2016 to 2021 in the USA. Emerg Med J [Internet]. 2024 [cited 2025 Jan 12];41(12). Available from: https://pubmed.ncbi.nlm.nih.gov/39375022/
14. Shalev A, Cho D, Marmar CR. Neurobiology and treatment of posttraumatic stress disorder. Am J Psychiatry. 2024;181(8):705–19.
15. Yoon S, Kim JE, Hwang J, Kang I, Jeon S, Im JJ, et al. Recovery from posttraumatic stress requires dynamic and sequential shifts in Amygdalar Connectivities. Neuropsychopharmacology [Internet] 2016 [cited 2025 Feb 9];42(2):454. Available from: https://pmc.ncbi.nlm.nih.gov/articles/PMC5399230/
16. Taylor KM, Thielking M, Mackelprang JL, Meyer D, Quinn S, Flatau P. When trauma violates trust: PTSD symptoms among chronically homeless adults in Australia. J Soc Distress Homeless. 2022;31(1):11–22.
17. Taylor KM, Thielking M, Mackelprang JL, Meyer D, Flatau P. Trauma involving violation of trust and mental health help seeking among homeless adults. Aust Psychol [Internet]. 2022 [cited 2024 Oct 6];57(3):174–85. Available from: https://www-tandfonline-com.proxy.bib.uottawa.ca/doi/abs/10.1080/00050067.2022.2059337
18. Classen CC, Palesh OG, Aggarwal R. Sexual revictimization: a review of the empirical literature. Trauma Violence Abuse [Internet] 2005 [cited 2025 May 3];6(2):103–129. Available from: https://pubmed.ncbi.nlm.nih.gov/15753196/
19. Levy MS. A helpful way to conceptualize and understand reenactments. J Psychother Pract Res. 1998;7(3):227–35. PMID: 9631344; PMCID: PMC3330499. https://pmc.ncbi.nlm.nih.gov/articles/PMC3330499/

20. Bowlby J. Attachment and loss: Volume 1 Attachment. Second. London, England: Penguin Books Ltd.; 1991.
21. Neves Horácio A, Bento A, Gama Marques J. Personality and attachment in the homeless: a systematic review. Int J Soc Psychiatry. 2023;69(6):1312–26.
22. Theodorou N, Johnsen S, Watts B, Burley A. Improving multiple exclusion homelessness (MEH) services: frontline worker responses to insecure attachment styles. J Mental Health Training Educat Pract. 2021;16(6):421–32.
23. Sochos A, Richards A, Smith S, Balint A, Bennett A. The attachment relationship between hostel-based homeless individuals and their keyworkers. Child Youth Serv Rev. 2023;149:106924.
24. Kozlowska K, Walker P, McLean L, Carrive P. Fear and the defense cascade: clinical implications and management. Harv Rev Psychiatry [Internet]. 2015 [cited 2025 Feb 12];23(4):263. Available from: https://pmc.ncbi.nlm.nih.gov/articles/PMC4495877/
25. Seigel DJ. The developing mind. 3rd ed. Guilford Press; 2020.
26. Ayano G, Solomon M, Tsegay L, Yohannes K, Abraha M. A systematic review and meta-analysis of the prevalence of post-traumatic stress disorder among homeless people. Psychiatry Q. 2020;91(4):949–63.
27. Armstrong R, Phillips L, Alkemade N, O'Donnell ML. Using latent class analysis to support the ICD-11 complex posttraumatic stress disorder diagnosis in a sample of homeless adults. J Trauma Stress [Internet] 2020 [cited 2024 Oct 6];33(5):677–687. Available from: https://onlinelibrary-wiley-com.proxy.bib.uottawa.ca/doi/full/10.1002/jts.22554
28. McQuillan K, Hyland P, Vallières F. Prevalence, correlates, and the mitigation of ICD-11 CPTSD among homeless adults: the role of self-compassion. Child Abuse Negl. 2022;127:105569.
29. Biskin RS. The lifetime course of borderline personality disorder. Can J Psychiatry [Internet] 2015 [cited 2024 Nov 12];60(7):303. Available from: https://pmc.ncbi.nlm.nih.gov/articles/PMC4500179/
30. Recommendations | Borderline personality disorder: recognition and management | Guidance | NICE [Internet]. [cited 2024 Nov 12]. Available from: https://www.nice.org.uk/guidance/cg78/chapter/Recommendations#assessment-and-management-by-community-mental-health-services
31. Weaver ICG, Cervoni N, Champagne FA, D'Alessio AC, Sharma S, Seckl JR, et al. Epigenetic programming by maternal behavior. Nat Neurosci [Internet]. 2004 Aug [cited 2024 Nov 3];7(8):847–54. Available from: https://pubmed.ncbi.nlm.nih.gov/15220929/
32. Housing, Infrastructure and Communities Canada – Homelessness Data Snapshot: The National Shelter Study 2021 Update [Internet]. [cited 2025 May 6]. Available from: https://housing-infrastructure.canada.ca/homelessness-sans-abri/reports-rapports/data-shelter-2021-donnees-refuge-eng.html

Trauma Informed Care

2

2.1 Trauma Informed Care Frameworks

A trauma-informed approach to care is not merely beneficial but essential, given the pervasive and often deeply rooted experiences of trauma that haunt many individuals grappling with homelessness. Trauma-informed care is a set of principles that aim to take into account people's experience of trauma, how it has affected them, how it may affect their relationships with potential carers, and how to design services to meet these needs. There is no single trauma-informed care model—a quick internet search reveals 4, 5, 6, or even 10 key principles of trauma-informed care. It is also notable that there is more written on the theory of trauma-informed care rather than how to operationalize it in different settings, especially in places where people who are homeless are likely to be seen. Also, much of the literature on trauma-informed care addresses what to do at an organizational level rather provide guidance to staff about what to do at a clinical level. However common threads include an emphasis on helping people feel safe, giving people choices, education on the effects of trauma, and focusing on strengths as well as difficulties (for a summary see Table 2.1). The often-stated approach is that trauma-informed care asks, "what happened to you" rather than "what is wrong with you." Reframing problems as a response to perceived danger caused by past experiences of trauma can generate novel ideas about how to help.

Modern approaches to trauma-informed care can be traced back to a series of seminal articles at the start of the millennium by Harris and Fallot [4] which described how they incorporated knowledge of trauma and its effects into their work in a traditional mental health setting in the US. The emphasis was on creating a trauma-informed service system, *"to be trauma informed means to know the history of past and current abuse in the life of the consumer with whom one is working. Such information allows for more holistic and integrated treatment planning. But second, and more important for this volume, to be trauma informed means to understand the role that violence and victimization play in the lives of most consumers of mental health and substance abuse services and to use that understanding to design*

S. Hatcher et al., *Street Mental Health Handbook*,
https://doi.org/10.1007/978-3-032-00663-9_2

Table 2.1 Summary of selected trauma-informed care frameworks

Principles	Description
Fallot and Harris (2009) Creating cultures of trauma-informed care [1]	
Safety	Promoting physical and emotional safety
Trustworthiness	Clear information about expectations, transitions, being patient and accepting
Choice	Being clear about options available
Collaboration	Seek feedback and acknowledge power dynamics
Empowerment	Build on strengths and identify personal goals
Hopper et al *(2010) Shelter from the storm; Trauma-informed care in homelessness services settings* [2]	
Trauma awareness	Recognising the impact of trauma
Safety	Physical and emotional safety
Choice and empowerment	Maximise choice
Strengths based	Instilling hope and building on strengths
SAMSHA (2014) Concept of trauma and guidance for a trauma-informed approach [3]	
Safety	Physical and psychological safety
Trustworthiness	Decisions are transparent to build trust
Peer support	Using peer support to establish safety and hope
Collaboration and mutuality	Power and decision making are shared
Empowerment voice and choice	Strengths and experiences are recognised and built upon
Cultural, historical and gender issues	Recognition and addressing of historical trauma

service systems that accommodate the vulnerabilities of trauma survivors and allow services to be delivered in a way that will facilitate consumer participation in treatment."

Trauma-informed care is not about trying to be friends with everyone and avoiding conflict. This may retraumatize people who experienced chaos and a lack of boundaries growing up. In trauma-informed care, establishing clear boundaries and consistent expectations is crucial for creating a sense of safety and predictability. This approach allows individuals to feel secure within a structured environment, which is particularly important for those who may have experienced unpredictability or instability in their past. By maintaining a balance between compassion and professionalism, caregivers can foster an atmosphere that promotes healing and personal growth.

2.2 Relational Mental Health

Trauma-informed care emphasizes the impact of trauma on patients' relationships, including those with caregivers. Individuals who have experienced abuse during childhood often learn that those who claim to care for them can cause harm, leading to significant trust issues. Consequently, building trust and fostering strong relationships with patients becomes crucial in engaging them and providing effective care.

The concept of "relational psychiatry" is relevant in this context, as it views the patient–caregiver relationship as a vital therapeutic tool and a catalyst for change. This approach assumes that the therapeutic relationship, or working alliance, is primarily responsible for improvement rather than any specific therapy. While substantial evidence supports this in psychotherapy settings, research in acute services outside formal psychotherapy is less extensive. Nevertheless, a meta-analysis [5] demonstrated that even in acute care settings, the quality of the therapeutic relationship significantly influences patient improvement. This finding underscores the importance of prioritizing relationship-building and trust development in trauma-informed care.

2.3 Clinical Trauma Informed Care with People Who Are Homeless

A systematic review examining the acceptability of health and social interventions for individuals experiencing homelessness identified recurring themes of marginalization, dehumanization, and exclusion from services [6]. Consequently, trust and personal safety were highly valued in interactions with health care providers.

> So, we don't adhere to street culture at all in the [safe consumption site] and that's why it can be a really safe space right? Because out there, there's the hierarchy … But we don't, we don't adhere to that at all, it, downstairs in the [safe consumption site] there's no outside talk a lot. Everyone needs to respect each other like… Any, any problems outside are left at the door so a lot of people find it's almost an escape for the hour that they're there. (Participant in [7])

A qualitative study [8] which asked people who were homeless what they needed from service providers to provide trauma-informed care found three themes. The first was that formal education and experience were important. This included knowledge about local services and a passion for the work. Second was the ability to build relationships to create trust. To do this, participants expected providers to be open about what they could or could not do, to check in regularly, to express concern for their health, to be consistent, to work with the same staff member and pay attention to privacy and confidentiality. The last was a theme around staff having supportive interpersonal styles. Staff could show this by being able to resolve conflict, offer care and support and understanding.

> … I found it can be really almost like shameful and debilitating to be working with a practitioner who has no sort of experience in what you're dealing with. It can be so hard to have to disclose information and you feel almost like you're talking to somebody who has like a degree and an education and everything and they know how to deal with it but you can feel almost judged or ashamed…I always feel more comfortable speaking to people who kind of have an understanding of what you're going through. (Participant in [7])

> Well, when a person's been traumatized, like their autonomy has been taken away, their voice has been taken away (long pause) …It's important to help them find their voice again. Have them speak… like determine… maybe they were in a situation where they were, they were gaslit, and they were told that their reality wasn't true, and so it's really important to give them that back like I hear you, I hear what you're saying, like thank you for your speaking truth, for you know, sharing, like being brave enough to share with me, things like that, and just create the safe space for them to be themselves again. (Participant in [7])

Appropriate self-disclosure can also help staff seem less “aloof” and “clinical.” One of us often introduces himself by explaining where his strange accent comes from and a bit about his background. He learnt this from working with Māori in New Zealand where introductions are always about trying to find connections before doing anything else.

> Honesty is the best policy … a lot of case managers and case workers say, “I had a rough night,” and I say, “Why? What happened?” They say, well, this and that and that and this, and then we get talking about that and talking about what’s happening with me, and then we look up it’s time go, you know, you like wow, thanks for sharing that with me ‘cuz I feel you human too. ‘Cuz you ain’t going to tell me you come in here every day with a shirt and tie on and everything been peachy cream. Sometimes you know. But the one’s say, um, “My profession tell me I cannot share that with you,” “Well, I don’t really need to talk to you, ‘cuz you’s a robot.” You know right now you telling cuz you that case manager and I the [participant], I cannot share certain thing with you. Well how can we ever get close? (Quoted in [8])

Often when people have been traumatized, they will defend themselves against being retraumatized by aggression, for example, by shouting, making threats or passively by retreating and not engaging. However, surviving and repairing these ruptures in relationships can be vital in building trust and developing self-esteem. Resolving conflict, which is a normal part of any relationship, with dignity and respect can be an important experience especially in those who have experienced conflict primarily through violence and humiliation. In one of our organizations, we share “country food” with clients, which helps to create a safe place:

> I think that one thing that I see that is always a hit is like country food days. Yeah, and I love it. It’s so sweet… And I’ve… you know, borne witness to so many of those country food days and it’s amazing just the, the level of community you know, like, you see all these people coming together and like eating together. It’s amazing. So, I think that absolutely, like food is a good incentive, but also like cultural food. (Participant in [7])

The relationship between a patient and clinician is a relationship like any other relationship. Key factors of good relationships are a lack of defensiveness, allowing yourself to be vulnerable, being curious, not making promises you can’t keep, and simply being kind. These can all play out in a clinical setting. When being criticized by a patient don’t be defensive. Be curious about what this means and where it comes from. Being vulnerable is often difficult for health care workers, but telling clients something about yourself is important and sometimes culturally necessary. Making promises and keeping them is important to gain trust so if you say you will see the patient in a week make sure that you do this. Being kind and compassionate may take many forms such as washing someone’s feet, getting them gloves, or a coffee. These acts can go a long way to building engagement. We have summarized clinical examples of trauma-informed care in Table 2.2.

Table 2.2 Clinical examples of trauma-informed care using the framework from Hopper [2]

Trauma awareness	If someone is aggressive towards you, don't be defensive or blame this on their "personality" but be curious why, acknowledging that people who have had a difficult start in life may have been hurt by people they trust and asking what might have happened to make them this way. Naming the "strong feeling in the room" (for example fear, anxiety, or anger) and linking it to a history of trauma Being honest about what you can and cannot provide (people facing homelessness have usually experienced rejection or "no" multiple times as well as unrealistic promises about what is available) Be knowledgeable about what community resources are available, for example, where can people get meals or help with identification documents. Have something to offer such as hand warmers, socks, or toiletries
Safety	No surprises—for example, preparing patients for staff changes or vacations (giving the gift of a "good ending") Letting people know who you are and who you work for. Interviewing people in safe places where you won't be interrupted or overheard. Being sensitive to social norms around eye contact, touch, and distance. Being clear what the rules are in the setting where you meet people (for example drug use, violence, acceptable behavior) Minimize potential triggers that may retraumatize people such as smells (often cleaning fluids in the settings where we work), sounds (sirens), or sights (flashing lights, uniforms). Having consistent routines for example always visiting a block, an encampment or a shelter at the same times each week. Be explicit and careful about privacy and confidentiality
Choice and empowerment	Asking the patient what they would like to get from the encounter Door open or closed and where would they like to sit (if seeing someone inside) Being clear they can end the encounter when they like but you'd be happy to see them again. Taking the time that is necessary rather than being dictated by clock time. Offering choices about treatment.
Strengths based	Acknowledging "transferrable skills," for example, drug dealers need to be able to "read" people, be good with figures, and manage multiple clients. Or that being in control and protecting others comes from growing up in an unpredictable often violent environment but could also be used to help others.

2.4 Balancing Care and Coercion

Despite the emphasis on trauma-informed care, there are times when clinicians will have to coerce people to do things they do not want to do. This often involves forcing them into hospital under mental health legislation. Obviously, this has the potential to retraumatize patients and damage relationships. The times when this is necessary usually involve when the patient is a significant threat to others or themselves. There are times when forcing someone into hospital can be the most compassionate thing to do, especially if someone is mentally ill and living in squalor with untreated health conditions without the capacity to make decisions about their health care. However, is it possible to forcibly hospitalize someone against their will in a trauma-informed way [9]? Good practice here involves trying all other options before forcing someone into hospital; trying to be clear about the process and the rights of the person; harm minimization of the process; being clear you will be there for them when they leave hospital; visiting them in hospital and liaising with the in-patient team. In our team after the person is discharged, we try to have a conversation with the patient about whether it was the right thing to do and what should we do differently in the future. The process of coercing care may also be helpful in synthesizing what we know about someone's condition and engaging others in care. In these circumstances, the clinicians can act as decision coordinator rather than decision maker [10].

Any decision-making about involuntary admissions also needs to take into account the longer term consequences of such a choice. A study in Demark followed 28 homeless patients who had been involuntarily hospitalized by an outreach psychiatric service in Copenhagen [11]. After a year 14 (50%) had a reduction of symptoms and 10 (36%) of the patients were taking antipsychotics. Another study in London, England, identified 32 people with psychosis who were homeless who had been admitted involuntarily and followed them up after 12 months [12]. Eighty percent were housed at 1 year and a similar proportion were in contact with a community mental health team.

2.5 Trauma-Informed Care at the Level of Organizations

Much more is written about trauma-informed care at an organizational level. The Substance Misuse and Mental Health Services Authority (SAMHSA) have developed a free Treatment Improvement Protocol (TIP) #57 on "Trauma-Informed Care in Behavioral Health Services" [13]. This document begins by describing the various types of trauma, their characteristics, and the factors that influence their impact. It underscores the importance of recognizing how widespread trauma is and its potential effects on individuals seeking behavioral health services. It includes the core principles for providing trauma-informed care within an organization including safety, trustworthiness, and transparency; peer support; collaboration and mutuality; Empowerment, Voice, and Choice; and Cultural, Historical, and Gender Considerations. The manual provides guidance on conducting thorough assessments that consider trauma history and its effects. It emphasizes the need for individualized treatment plans that incorporate trauma-informed strategies to support recovery. It also highlights the importance of training and supporting health professionals to adopt a trauma-informed approach. This includes ongoing education, supervision, and self-care practices to prevent secondary traumatic stress and burnout among providers. Also, SAMHSA's TIP55 "Behavioral Health Services for People who are Homeless" [14] provides guidance on addressing needs in this population. It emphasizes the need for integrated trauma-informed approaches and the necessity of addressing both housing and treatment needs concurrently for effective interventions.

A more recent development has been the development of "Psychologically Informed Environments" (PIE) [15]. The components of psychologically informed environments include:

A Psychological framework: This helps services understand and respond to the people they support
Physical environment: Considers how the physical space affects people
Staff training: Helps staff support people's psychological needs
Relationships: Focuses on building relationships with people
Evidence generation: Evaluates the outcomes of services

The difference between services that are trauma informed and those that are psychologically informed environments is largely one of semantics. However, in theory those services that are trauma informed explicitly adopt a trauma theory and awareness model, whereas those that are psychologically informed environments use a broader range of psychological frameworks. Homeless Link in England provides a summary of trauma-informed care and psychologically informed environments [16] as well as guidance on reflective practice, avoiding vicarious trauma and other resources for organizations [17].

In practice, one of the skills of clinical work is knowing which way of thinking generates the most useful solutions for the person in front of you. Thinking biologically and using the DSM V framework maybe very useful seeing someone who is delirious or psychotic, whereas thinking psychodynamically may be helpful in explaining complex life experiences including repeated patterns that keep individuals trapped in their trauma.

References

1. Fallot RD, Harris M. Creating cultures of trauma-informed care (CCTIC): a self-assessment and planning protocol. Washington, DC: Community Connections; 2009.
2. Hopper EK, Bassuk EL, Olivet J. Shelter from the storm: trauma-informed care in homelessness services settings. Open Health Serv Policy J [Internet]. 2010;2:131–51. Available from: http://www.traumacenter.org/products/pdf_files/shelter_from_storm.pdf.
3. Substance Abuse and Mental Health Services Administration. SAMHSA's Concept of trauma and guidance for a trauma-informed approach. HHS Publication No. (SMA) 14-4884. Rockville: Substance Abuse and Mental Health Services Administration; 2014.
4. Harris M, Fallot RD. Envisioning a trauma-informed service system: a vital paradigm shift. New Dir Ment Health Serv. 2001;(89):3–22.
5. Martin DJ, Garske JP, Katherine DM. Relation of the therapeutic alliance with outcome and other variables: a meta-analytic review. J Consult Clin Psychol. 2000;68(3):438–50.
6. Magwood O, Leki VY, Kpade V, Saad A, Alkhateeb Q, Gebremeskel A, et al. Common trust and personal safety issues: a systematic review on the acceptability of health and social interventions for persons with lived experience of homelessness. PLoS One. 2019;14(12):e0226306.
7. Edgar N, Maclean S, Jormand M, Paranjkhoo P, Hatcher, S. Designing a trauma informed service to deliver traumatherapy with people experiencing homelessness: a qualitative study. BMC Health Services Research; 2025 (In Press). https://doi.org/10.1186/s12913-025-13428-8

8. Barry AR, Hoffman E, Martinez-Charleston E, Demario M, Stewart J, Mohiuddin M, et al. Trauma-informed interactions within a trauma-informed homeless service provider: staff and client perspectives. J Community Psychol. 2024;52(2):415–34.
9. Rosenbaum L. Liberty versus need — our struggle to care for people with serious mental illness. N Engl J Med [Internet]. 2016 [cited 2025 Feb 23];375(15):1490–5. Available from: https://www-nejm-org.proxy.bib.uottawa.ca/doi/full/10.1056/NEJMms1610124.
10. Trestman RL, Nagaraja K. Case and commentary: peer-reviewed article how should clinicians execute critical force interventions with compassion, not just harm minimization, as a clinical and ethical goal? AMA J Ethics. 2021;23(4):292–7.
11. Frisk Vorting A, Gram Henriksen M, Nordgaard J. Changes in clinical and social situation after involuntary admission of homeless people with psychotic disorders: a one-year follow-up study. Nord J Psychiatry. ISSN: (Print). 2021 [cited 2025 Jan 28]. Available from: https://www.tandfonline.com/action/journalInformation?journalCode=ipsc20ARTICLE.
12. Timms P, Perry J. Involuntary admission to hospital of homeless people with schizophrenia from the street – 1 year outcomes. Eur Psychiatry. 2015;30:900.
13. (US) C for SAT. Trauma-Informed Care in Behavioral Health Services [Internet]. Substance Abuse and Mental Health Services Administration (US); 2014 [cited 2025 May 3]. Available from: https://www.ncbi.nlm.nih.gov/books/NBK207201/.
14. TIP 55: behavioral health services for people who are homeless | SAMHSA [Internet]. [cited 2025 May 3]. Available from: https://www.samhsa.gov/resource/dbhis/tip-55-behavioral-health-services-people-who-are-homeless.
15. Psychologically informed services for homeless people. Good Practice Guide [Internet]. 2012 [cited 2025 May 3]. Available from: https://tinyurl.com/yfzttfsr.
16. Trauma-informed care and psychologically informed environments | Homeless Link [Internet]. [cited 2025 May 3]. Available from: https://homeless.org.uk/knowledge-hub/trauma-informed-care-and-psychologically-informed-environments/.
17. Reflective practice in homelessness services | Homeless Link [Internet]. [cited 2025 May 3]. Available from: https://homeless.org.uk/knowledge-hub/reflective-practice-in-homelessness-services/.

Assessment of Mental Disorders

3

3.1 Introduction

The chaos of the streets and competing priorities of people sleeping rough often leave limited time for mental health assessments, which, when performed the way in which public insurance requires and psychiatric residents are taught, can take an hour to an hour and a half. A good street-based mental health assessment should be brief and respectful of the person's time. In order to maximize value and minimize time, assessments should aim to answer two questions within 10 to 15 min: "What do I need to know to prescribe medication?" and "What do I need to know to reduce safety risks?" When on the streets, mental health assessments should aim at treating *symptom clusters*, rather than specific *diagnoses*. A good-enough diagnosis, or a "street diagnosis," is more important than a perfect diagnosis. This chapter introduces the Rapid Street Psych Assessment, developed to differentiate between symptoms of various common psychiatric diagnoses among people sleeping rough with cooccurring substance use disorders.

3.2 First, Build Trust

As an essential component of working with people sleeping rough, building trust is far more important than making a diagnosis. Trauma, as described in previous chapters, is universal among people sleeping outside and trauma from previous psychiatric treatment is common. Because of these traumatic experiences, people sleeping rough often fear discussions about mental health concerns. For many people living outside, their only interactions with psychiatrists before have been in involuntary settings. In order to promote healing and well-being, clinicians must work hard to make street-based evaluations and treatment a completely different experience. The experience should be filled with choice, respect, autonomy, and patient-led goal-making with a treatment provider who is transparent, authentic, and keeps their promises.

S. Hatcher et al., *Street Mental Health Handbook*,
https://doi.org/10.1007/978-3-032-00663-9_3

Before starting an evaluation, I offer reassurance that an assessment is really only an assessment with no strings attached. I tell patients that if I think treatment can help, I will offer it, but that I will never force it and I will never make them take a medication they hate. I say, "it's your body and you decide what goes into it." I explain that an assessment helps us both understand what is happening with a person's brain and body. A mental health diagnosis can help the person qualify for specific housing options and make a successful claim for government benefits, even if the person is uninterested in treatment.

Once the person feels sufficiently comfortable, begin the evaluation. Keep in mind that some patients may not trust you enough to start an assessment for many months of informal street visits. Others may agree to an assessment only because they have no other viable options for mental health treatment. It is our job, as street medicine professionals, to demonstrate that we are trustworthy at every opportunity.

3.3 The Order of Assessment with the RSPA

The order of questions in the RSPA, which can be found in Fig. 3.1, is intentional and focused on two concepts. First, prescribing *only* an antidepressant to someone with psychosis or bipolar disorder is harmful because it can worsen psychosis or cause mania. Therefore, the first two steps of the RSPA focus on ruling in or out psychosis and a history of mania. The second concept helps with reducing the time it takes to make a street diagnosis and prescribe medication. For instance, if you know the person is having hallucinations, you know they need an antipsychotic. You may observe some people responding to the hallucinations or delusions without asking any questions; this makes for an incredibly fast assessment. If you know the

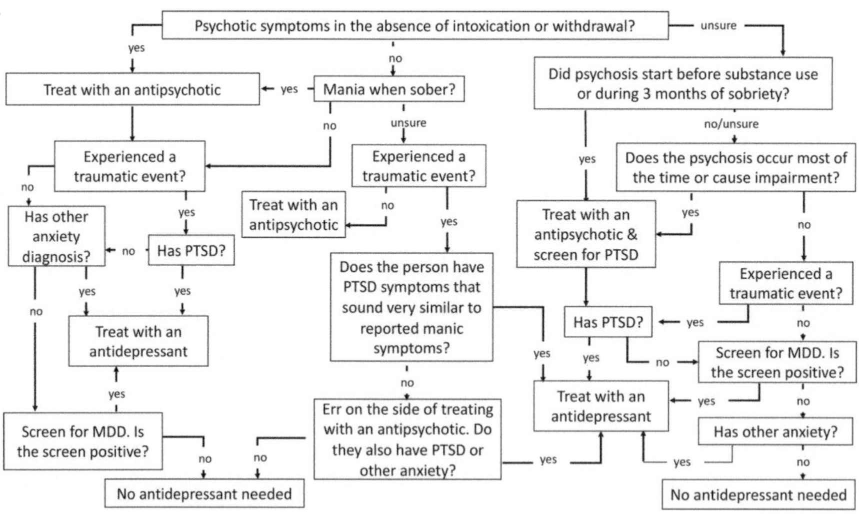

Fig. 3.1 The Rapid Street Psych Assessment

person needs an antipsychotic, you do not need to evaluate for a history of mania because an antipsychotic will treat bipolar disorder. Bipolar disorder is more difficult to diagnose than psychosis, which is why assessing for psychosis is prioritized.

If you rule out psychosis, the RSPA guides you to evaluate for a history of mania next. If positive, you do not need to assess symptoms of depression (except for suicidal ideation) because you can safely assume that if a person has manic episodes they will also have depressive episodes. Additionally, antipsychotics act to stabilize mood, meaning that it treats both the bipolar depression and mania. You may know that some antipsychotics are approved by the United States (U.S.) Food and Drug Administration (FDA) solely for bipolar mania or bipolar depression, but in practice antipsychotics are used to treat both.

Once psychosis and mania are ruled out, assess for post-traumatic stress disorder (PTSD). PTSD is more common than depression among people sleeping rough and diagnosing depression can be challenging for people living on the streets. If you assess for depression first, you still need to assess for PTSD, whereas if you know the person has PTSD and prescribe an antidepressant, it will also treat depression if it exists.

Anytime you determine the correct medication to prescribe during the RSPA, you can stop the diagnostic assessment, particularly if time is limited. Over the next several visits, you should still assess for symptoms of other mental health diagnoses because you will gain a better sense of the total burden of symptoms as well as knowledge of symptoms to monitor. In bipolar disorder, for example, you may be able to prevent manic episodes with a lower antipsychotic dose, but you may need to increase the dose to effectively treat the depression symptoms.

While the RSPA guides clinicians towards a street mental health diagnosis and appropriate medication treatment, you will still need to perform other parts of a brief but thorough assessment. At minimum, document allergies, other health conditions, and a list of current medications to ensure safe prescribing.

3.4 Evaluating for Psychosis in the Absence of Substance Intoxication or Withdrawal

Psychosis is often described as losing touch with reality. More obvious symptoms include delusions and/or hallucinations (auditory, visual, tactile, or olfactory), and disorganized speech and thoughts. Less obvious symptoms include withdrawal from others, minimal speech, self-neglect, amotivation, and anhedonia. Though there are many psychiatric diagnoses that include psychosis, the DSM-5-TR criteria for schizophrenia and schizoaffective disorders are listed below. Psychotic symptoms are typically treated with antipsychotics and with the time limitations inherent to many street encounters, diagnostic criteria are less important than symptom recognition with the RSPA.

Because many substances cause psychotic symptoms, it is helpful to tease apart the substance use from the psychotic symptoms when possible. If a person only has psychotic symptoms during intoxication or withdrawal, they may not need daily antipsychotic treatment. At times, though, a dose or two of antipsychotic can help to reduce psychosis during intoxication or withdrawal when needed. For example, a man having scary hallucinations while withdrawing from crack would benefit from a supply of several doses of an antipsychotic. A daily antipsychotic typically helps people who frequently have psychotic symptoms, even if you suspect the psychosis is solely caused by the substance. If a person uses less or stops using, you can always reassess the need for a daily antipsychotic. See the chapter on substance use disorders for details about effects, side effects, and treatment of various substances.

You can either assess for psychosis first or substance use first. If the person has obvious psychotic symptoms, you do not need to ask questions about psychosis; you only need to ask about substance use. Otherwise, the following exchange between you (dashed line) and your new friend, Baby E (solid line) in Fig. 3.2, can be helpful in initiating the assessment:

Given that Baby E continued to have auditory hallucinations after 2 months of no substance use, treatment with an antipsychotic medication is warranted, particularly if the symptoms are bothersome or interfere with functioning. Though methamphetamine use can cause hallucinations for months or longer, if the symptoms are daily or bothersome enough, an antipsychotic can be helpful. Baby E does not necessarily need to take antipsychotics for life, however, as symptoms can abate. When Baby E is in a more stable living situation, such as living in a safe indoor environment, or not using drugs for more than two months, she may no longer have hallucinations.

It is important to keep in mind that there are hallucinations that occur in people without psychosis. Hearing sounds that occur only when asleep, falling asleep, or just waking up are not hallucinations that need treatment. Similarly, it may be culturally appropriate for people to see or hear deceased loved ones. For these situations, ask the patient if they have family or friends who have these experiences as well, which would suggest a culturally normative experience rather than symptoms of a psychotic illness. Equally, if the experience is more like a memory of the person who died, the person likely does not have a psychotic illness.

It is also important to recognize the role racism plays in biasing our diagnoses. In both the United States and Canada, Black people are diagnosed with schizophrenia far more often that White people. This difference is not due to differences in the prevalence of schizophrenia between Black and White people; rather it is a difference rooted in the racial bias of a predominantly White mental health workforce. When performing a mental health evaluation, take extra care to discern if PTSD, bipolar disorder, severe grief, or other factors are the cause of symptoms among your Black patients.

If Baby E denied ever having hallucinations, asking about delusions is next. "Have you ever believed something, but other people didn't think it was real. Or have you ever thought people were following you or out to get you?" The more improbable the answer, the more likely the thought is delusional. Examples include, "the FBI follows me everywhere I go" or "I can tell she is filming me everywhere

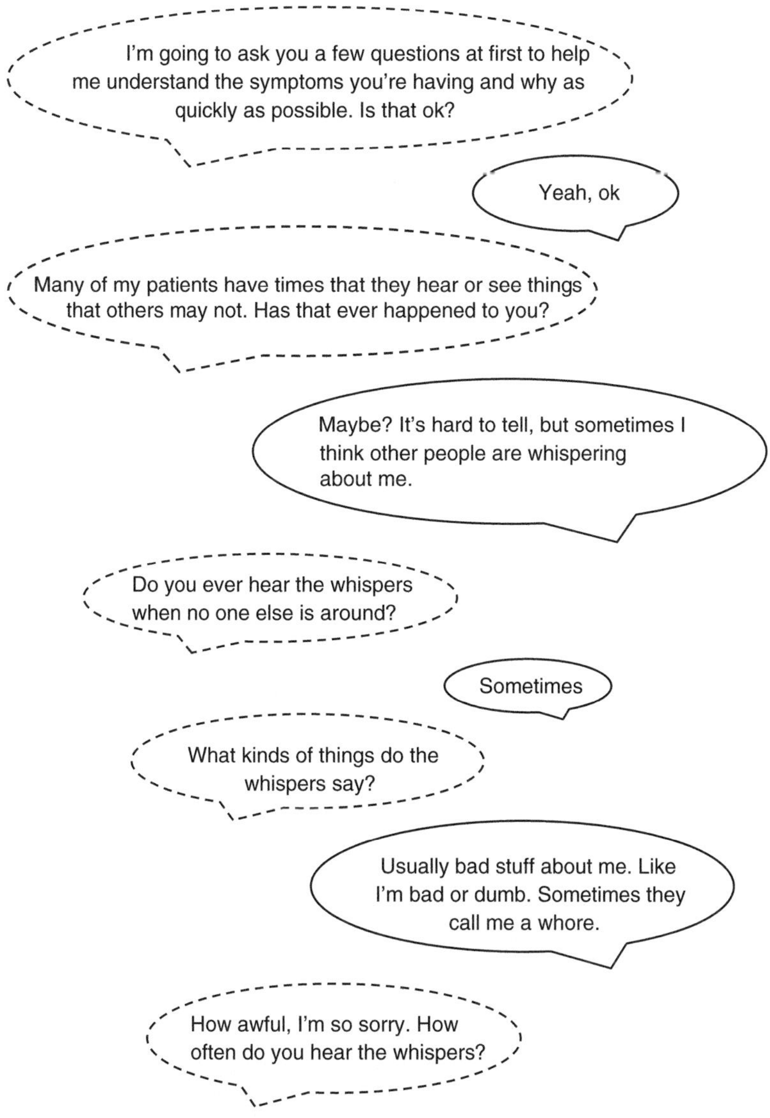

Fig. 3.2 Assessment for psychosis

because I see that red laser beam, even in my apartment when I had one. Even in the bathroom." It would also be reasonable to ask at some point if she has ever seen a psychiatrist, whether she wanted to or not, and ask what the psychiatrist's diagnosis was. However, psychiatrists are humans and incorrectly diagnose patients at times; it is always best to ask your own questions too.

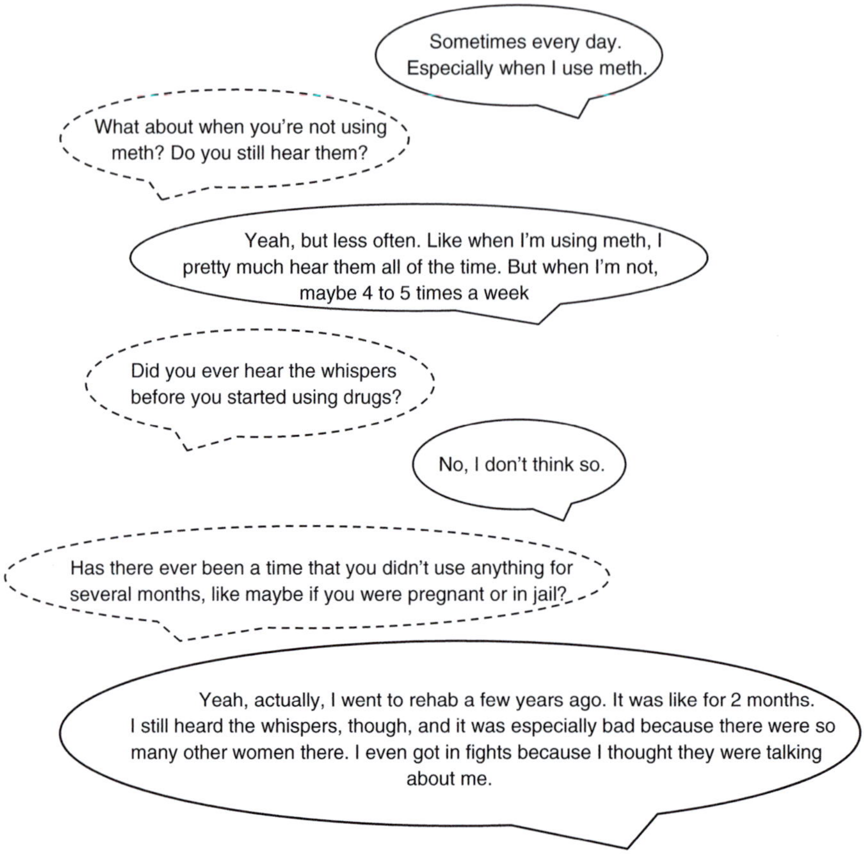
Sometimes every day. Especially when I use meth.
What about when you're not using meth? Do you still hear them?
Yeah, but less often. Like when I'm using meth, I pretty much hear them all of the time. But when I'm not, maybe 4 to 5 times a week
Did you ever hear the whispers before you started using drugs?
No, I don't think so.
Has there ever been a time that you didn't use anything for several months, like maybe if you were pregnant or in jail?
Yeah, actually, I went to rehab a few years ago. It was like for 2 months. I still heard the whispers, though, and it was especially bad because there were so many other women there. I even got in fights because I thought they were talking about me.

Fig. 3.2 (continued)

Differentiating Between Psychosis and Post-traumatic Stress Disorder (PTSD)

Questions about delusions can be tricky, especially when the person also has PTSD. If you are unsure, go ahead and ask about trauma, even though the trauma assessment is lower in the order of questions in the RSPA. Questions such as, "Have you ever had anything bad happen to you, being beaten or raped, shot at, anything like that?" can help distinguish between a paranoid delusion and fear secondary to trauma. If Baby E answered yes, follow up with "Is that the person you're worried is following you?" If she answers yes again, PTSD is more likely the cause of her experience as opposed to psychosis. Equally, people with PTSD can hear or see things others cannot during a flashback (an experience of re-living the traumatic event). People with PTSD may sometimes hear their name being called, even when they are alone or feel someone touching them. These symptoms usually do not require antipsychotic medication, as they usually abate with antidepressants and/or therapy. Rarely, with treatment-persistent symptoms, antipsychotics have been used with success in PTSD treatment.

3.5 Substance Use Assessment

If you start your conversation with Baby E asking about psychotic symptoms, you still need to assess substance use, as drugs and alcohol can also mimic manic symptoms. Assume that people use drugs and alcohol, homeless or not, and ask questions accordingly. In order to maintain trust during this conversation, use a very nonjudgmental approach. Prefacing the conversation about substances can also help. "I ask questions about substance use for everyone because it's helpful for me to do a faster assessment this way." Or, "Alcohol and drugs can sometimes make it seem like you have a mental health diagnosis even when you don't."

You only need to do a good-enough substance use history modified for the streets. You likely do not have time to ask all questions for all drugs. Asking about their favorite substance or the one they use most, how much and how often, can make the evaluation faster. Then, you may also ask, "What other drugs have you ever used?" If the person reports none, a good response is, "None? Really, never ever?" If their preferred drug is one that does not usually cause psychosis, you should also ask about methamphetamine and cocaine. The following dialogue in Fig. 3.3 between you (dashed line) and Baby E (solid line), may help you assess substance use.

For someone who uses drugs most of the time and has psychotic symptoms, it can be unclear if the psychosis would stop in the absence of drug use. Rarely are people able to stop using substances entirely or for a sustained amount of time while living on the streets; expecting them to quit using in such a chaotic environment will only frustrate you and your friends sleeping unsheltered. If the person is experiencing psychotic symptoms often enough to be bothersome or to impair functioning, err on the side of treating with antipsychotics. You can—and should—always reassess your street diagnosis and medication treatment, when the situation changes.

In the RSPA, any time the decision tree leads to treating with an antipsychotic, you can stop the assessment if desired because you know what medication you are going to prescribe first. On the streets, antipsychotics are usually the safest choice for treating Bipolar disorder. If a person has psychotic symptoms, you do not need to know if they have ever had mania. Though there are subsequent questions in the RSPA to assess for PTSD and depression, you are not required to evaluate for every disorder during the first visit.

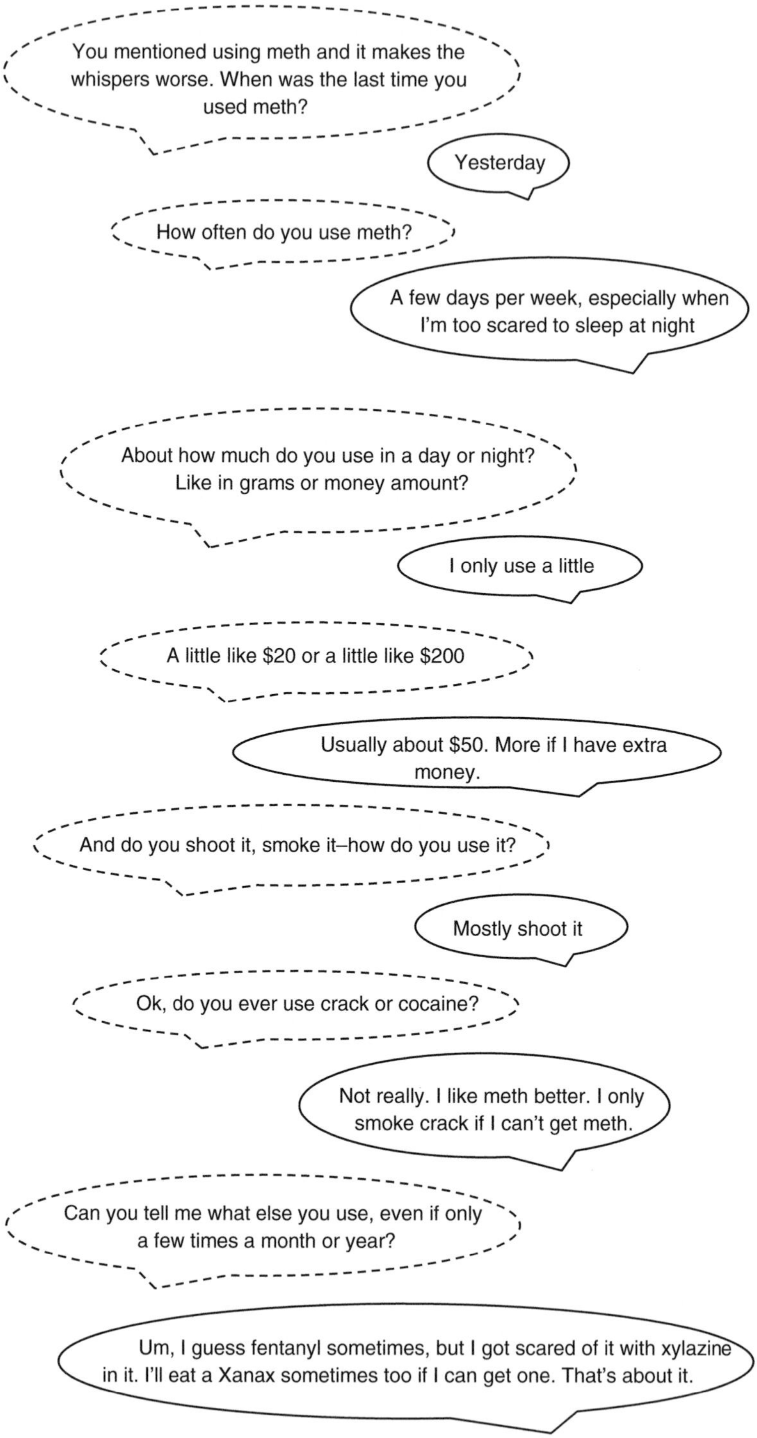

Fig. 3.3 Assessment for substance use

3.6 Assessment for a History of Mania

In the absence of psychotic symptoms, assessing for a history of mania is the next order of business in the RSPA. Patients are rarely experiencing a manic episode at the time of the assessment; evaluating for a *history* of mania is important. Mania is characterized by moods of euphoria and/or excessive irritability and cannot be diagnosed in the absence of these mood symptoms. Additional symptoms of mania include decreased need for sleep (not decreased ability to sleep), rapid speech or talking much more than usual, distractibility, grandiosity, and psychomotor agitation. Some people have grandiose or paranoid delusions with mania or irritable or euphoric auditory hallucinations.

Many clinicians may be familiar with and find the mnemonic DIGFAST helpful to remember the symptoms of mania. DIGFAST stands for **D**istractibility, **I**rritability, **G**randiosity, **F**light of ideas, **A**ctivity increase, **S**leep deficit, and **T**alkativeness. For the purposes of the RSPA, you do not need to distinguish between mania and hypomania. If the person, during the absence of substance use, had euphoria and three additional symptoms, or irritability and four other symptoms, lasting for four or more days, mania is probable. Ideally, you would ask determine if the person had these symptoms during a period of sobriety lasting three or more months.

If the person is willing to complete a questionnaire and you have someone on hand who can read it to them if they prefer, you can use the Mood Disorder Questionnaire (MDQ) to assist in the diagnosis. The MDQ is freely available online. Preface the questionnaire by telling the person to only think of a time when they had not used drugs or alcohol in at least a month. If you know the criteria for mania, however, the following conversation between you (dashed line) and Cowboy (solid line) in Fig. 3.4 will take less time than performing the MDQ. The words in brackets indicate the symptom you're evaluating.

In the conversation above, Cowboy reports many symptoms of mania and appears to have met criteria for previous manic episodes. He notes four or more days of irritability with at least four additional symptoms: increased energy, increased goal-directed activity, racing thoughts, decreased need for sleep, and pleasurable activities with painful consequences.

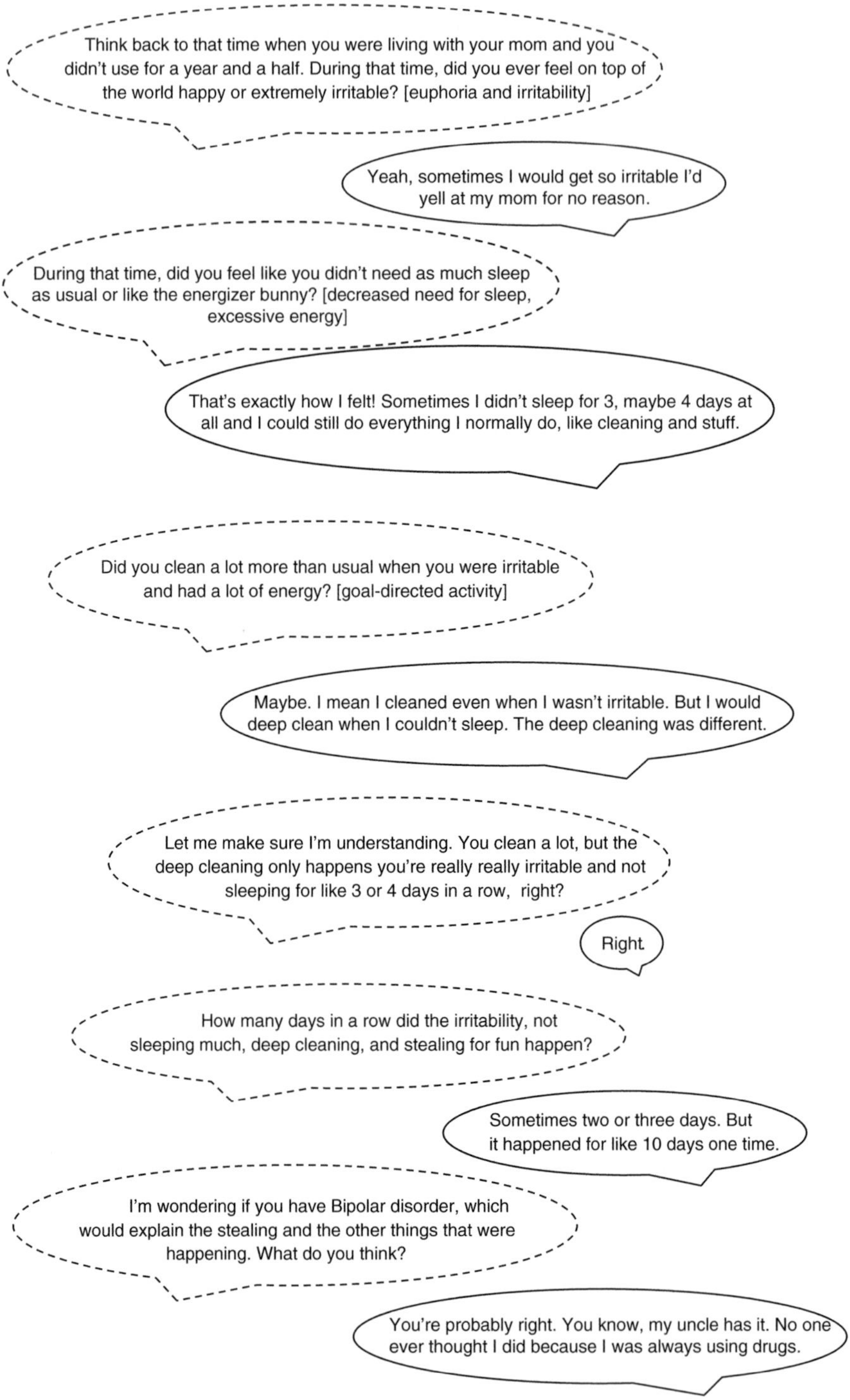
Think back to that time when you were living with your mom and you didn't use for a year and a half. During that time, did you ever feel on top of the world happy or extremely irritable? [euphoria and irritability]
Yeah, sometimes I would get so irritable I'd yell at my mom for no reason.
During that time, did you feel like you didn't need as much sleep as usual or like the energizer bunny? [decreased need for sleep, excessive energy]
That's exactly how I felt! Sometimes I didn't sleep for 3, maybe 4 days at all and I could still do everything I normally do, like cleaning and stuff.
Did you clean a lot more than usual when you were irritable and had a lot of energy? [goal-directed activity]
Maybe. I mean I cleaned even when I wasn't irritable. But I would deep clean when I couldn't sleep. The deep cleaning was different.
Let me make sure I'm understanding. You clean a lot, but the deep cleaning only happens you're really really irritable and not sleeping for like 3 or 4 days in a row, right?
Right
How many days in a row did the irritability, not sleeping much, deep cleaning, and stealing for fun happen?
Sometimes two or three days. But it happened for like 10 days one time.
I'm wondering if you have Bipolar disorder, which would explain the stealing and the other things that were happening. What do you think?
You're probably right. You know, my uncle has it. No one ever thought I did because I was always using drugs.

Fig. 3.4 Assessment for mania

3.7 Going Down the Rabbit Hole

If you have heard the diagnoses Bipolar I and Bipolar II, do not worry about distinguishing between the two with the Rapid Street Psych Evaluation, as both diagnoses are treated with the same medications on the streets. For those who are interested in the difference, an episode of mania requires that symptoms last seven or more days, or at least four days requiring either concurrent psychosis or hospitalization for the episode. If a person has ever had a manic episode, diagnose Bipolar I. For Bipolar II, the person can only ever have had hypomanic episodes. The same DIGFAST symptoms should be present in hypomanic episodes, but they last at least four but no more than six days. The DSM classifies hospitalization and/or psychotic symptoms during an episode as mania instead of hypomania, even if the episode only lasted four to six days. Table 3.1 below shows the difference between mood disorders and psychotic disorders of different types based on symptoms. While it can be helpful to understand the criteria for the different diagnoses below, all of the diagnoses except Major Depressive Disorder (MDD) *without* psychosis are treated with antipsychotics in the street setting. MDD is the only diagnosis treated with antidepressants alone in Table 3.1.

Further criteria distinguishing between the diagnosis are irrelevant (and likely antithetical) to making a rapid street diagnosis and do not affect treatment decisions in the street-based setting. Please refer to the Diagnostic and Statistical Manual 5th edition (DSM V) or texts about psychiatric diagnostic assessments if you would like additional information. Note that the further you pursue an exactly correct diagnosis in the street medicine setting, the more likely it is that you will take too long to come to a medication treatment decision. More lengthy diagnostic evaluations typically result in the patient becoming frustrated or annoyed that you do not value their time or understand their competing needs. The longer you take to make an exact diagnosis instead of a good-enough diagnosis, the less time you will have to diagnose and treat other patients on the street. Because there are so few physicians and advance

Table 3.1 Differentiating symptoms of mood and psychotic disorders

	MDD	MDD with psychotic features	Bipolar II	Bipolar I	SCAD[a] depressed type	SCAD[a] bipolar type	Schizophrenia
Depressive episode	+	+	±	±	+	±	±
Hypomanic episode	–	–	+	±	–	N/A	–
Manic episode	–	–	–	+	–	+	–
Psychotic symptoms	–	+	–	±	+	+	+

[a]Schizoaffective Disorder

+ indicates the episode or symptoms are required for the diagnosis; – indicates the episode or symptoms to be absent to make the diagnosis; ± indicates the episode or symptoms may or may not be present, but they are not required to make the diagnosis; “a” indicates Schizoaffective disorder practice providers (APP) willing or able to treat mental illness on the streets, taking this public mental health approach can help you do the most good for the most people.

Diagnostic assessments are important and should be performed, but they should not unnecessarily prevent or delay medication treatment. And, if you come to the wrong diagnostic conclusion, the benefit of street medicine is seeing the patient frequently and being able to reevaluate and change treatment plans quickly. Psychiatrists in offices make mistakes in diagnosis too, but if they are limited to seeing the patient every three months or even every month, treatment of an incorrect diagnosis may continue for longer than an incorrect diagnosis in the street medicine setting.

3.8 Assessment for Post-traumatic Stress Disorder (PTSD)

Next in the order of the Rapid Street Psych Assessment is PTSD, as it is likely the most widespread anxiety disorder among people sleeping rough. Because the RSPA focuses on determining which medication to use in the shortest amount of time, screening for a common diagnosis treated with antidepressants is a fast method for determining if an antidepressant is warranted. Screening for further diagnoses treated by antidepressants is unnecessary once the PTSD diagnosis is a made, as the antidepressant will treat any of those other diagnoses as well.

PTSD is a very frequent cause of distress, anxiety, fluctuating emotions, and angry outbursts that may be reported to you. The pooled prevalence of PTSD in a 2020 meta-analysis of people who are homeless in seven countries was 27.38%, though individual studies included varied from 1.89% to 78.57% [1]. The fluctuating emotions and angry outbursts are commonly misattributed to Bipolar disorder by patients, families, homeless service agency staff, and others. While the extreme anxiety and mistrust related to PTSD can cause people to sleep outside as opposed to sleeping in a shelter, their angry outbursts may result in being kicked out of or banned from shelters. Accurately evaluating and treating PTSD can result in improved ability to tolerate and not be removed from shared living environments. PTSD has numerous symptoms and making a diagnosis on the streets can be time-consuming.

Rather than memorize and ask patients about each symptom, the PTSD Checklist for DSM-5 (PCL-5) is a 20-item evidence-based questionnaire developed by staff at the United States Department of Veterans Affairs National Center for PTSD. A military version based on the DSM-IV-TR, called the "PCL-M" is a 17-item questionnaire that can be used instead for veterans with stressful military experiences, though the PCL-5 will likely suffice for all patients. The checklist is a public domain document and can be accessed freely online. If your medical record has a PCL-5 form, it may be helpful to input the answers there to track score changes over time.

Before having a person complete the questionnaire, asking about traumatic experiences is very helpful because the PCL-5 only refers to them as "stressful experiences." Otherwise, your patient may have a false negative or positive screen for PTSD. Try to be thorough, but quick in screening for trauma. You may tell patients you do not need to know what the trauma was, just that they had the trauma. Rattle off the following: "Have you ever had anything really horrible happen to you? You don't have to tell me about it if you don't want to, but it's helpful to know—yes or no—if you've been had any of these things happen to you or if you've seen them happen to others. Have you ever been in a natural disaster, flood, or fire; been threatened with a weapon, physically harmed in any way, being verbally or emotionally harmed; sexually harmed; been bullied in school; witnessed someone die, seen a dead body, seen someone overdose; been in combat in the military; in a horrible car accident; kidnapped or held hostage. Have you ever seen any of these things happen to other people?" If they say no to all of these, try a few more questions: "Have you ever been in jail or prison and seen horrible things happen to someone? Have you ever been in solitary confinement?" or "What about how you ended up on the streets?"

The other questions you may ask before using the PCL-5—because a 20-item questionnaire is long for patients to complete—is "Do you ever have nightmares about the bad things that happened, feel like you're reliving it, have memories of it suddenly that you don't want?" If the answer is yes to any kind of trauma and nightmares, flashbacks, and unwanted memories, the PCL-5 is worth completing. Offer to have someone on the team read it to them; if they can read well, they usually say they can complete it themselves. Tell them that when the questionnaire says "stressful experience," think of the bad things we just talked about.

Scoring and interpretation information is provided with the checklist. Scoring ranges from zero to 80 and a score of 70 or 80 is unsurprising for people living unsheltered. A PCL-5 score of 31–33 is recommended as a cut-off point; the PCL-5 authors report that this score indicates probable PTSD. For the purposes of the Rapid Street Psych Assessment, a probable diagnosis is sufficient. Occasionally, someone who has PTSD may score less than 30, but have a high score on avoidance symptoms. Because avoidance symptoms cause the person to avoid all thoughts and feelings associated with their trauma, the PCL-5 will be falsely low. People who frequently use opioids or drugs to help them avoid memories, thoughts, and feelings related to their trauma may also have a falsely low score. In these cases, keep PTSD in your differential diagnosis and occasionally reevaluate for PTSD, as an individual's ability to avoid thoughts and feelings can be challenging in the stressful setting of the streets.

3.9 Differentiating Between Mania, ADHD, and PTSD

Returning to Cowboy, he also mentions ADHD, which can cause diagnostic confusion. To assist with diagnostic clarification, the Venn diagram in Fig. 3.5 shows symptoms of mania, ADHD, and PTSD that overlap and those that are unique to each diagnosis. Given these overlaps, it is easy to see how a patient could be misdiagnosed. People on the streets have often been misdiagnosed with Bipolar disorder—either by psychiatry, others, or themselves—when they actually have PTSD, ADHD, substance use disorders, or all of the above. Be skeptical of a diagnosis of

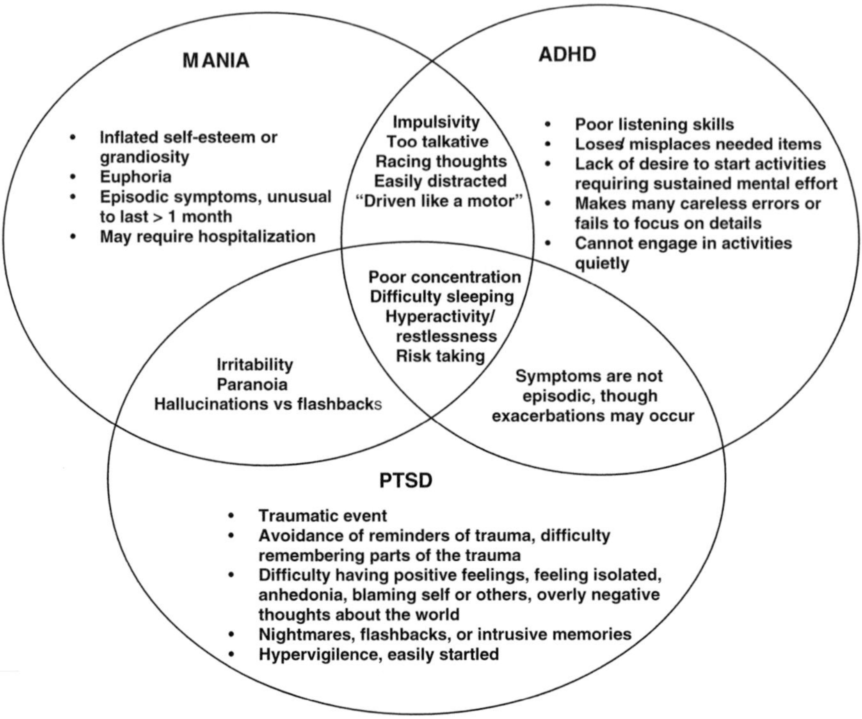

Fig. 3.5 Characteristics of mania, ADHD, and PTSD

Bipolar disorder in a person's chart if the chart does not clearly document the person's symptoms of mania. You may often find yourself "un-diagnosing" Bipolar disorder for people sleeping unsheltered and diagnosing PTSD, which is surprisingly under-diagnosed among this population.

3.10 Assessment for Other Anxiety Disorders

If the patient's main complaint is anxiety, but they do not meet criteria for PTSD, you may need to ask screening questions about a few other anxiety disorders. To cover the bases, ask questions in Table 3.2 below about Generalized Anxiety Disorder (GAD), Obsessive Compulsive Disorder (OCD), and Panic Disorder.

There are screening tools listed in Table 3.3 for each of these disorders, if needed, though their usefulness on the streets is questionable. People sleeping outside commonly have PTSD. If you know they have PTSD, you do not need to know if they have another anxiety disorder; the anxiety disorders are all treated the same—with an antidepressant. That being said, if the patient continues to report extreme anxiety despite adequate treatment for PTSD, suspect OCD.

Table 3.2 Screening questions for GAD, OCD, and panic disorder

Diagnosis	Key words	Question
GAD	"Worry"	Do you find yourself *worrying* most of the time, maybe more than you think you should?
OCD	"Over and over"	Is there anything you do *over and over and over*, like washing your hands or body, counting things, arranging things, going through things you said in the day to find something wrong?
Panic disorder	"Suddenly"	Do you *suddenly* find yourself really anxious for no reason? What does it feel like physically?

Table 3.3 Questionnaires for GAD, OCD, and panic disorder

Diagnosis	Tool	Details
GAD	GAD-7	Interpretation of score: 0–4 minimal anxiety; 5–9 mild anxiety, 10–14 moderate anxiety; >15 severe anxiety
OCD	Y-BOCS	Use the 10-item questionnaire. The symptom checklist is helpful, but supplementary Interpretation of score: 0–7 nonclinical; 8–15 mild; 16–23 moderate; 24–31 severe; 32–40 extreme https://pandasnetwork.org/wp-content/uploads/2018/11/y-bocs-w-checklist.pdf
Panic	PHQ-PD	Scoring: each "yes" answer counts as 1 point Interpretation: 5 or more points is suggestive of panic disorder

3.11 Assessment for Major Depressive Disorder

Screening for depression is the final official step in the RSPA. If a person on the street comes to you with concern for depression, you may skip screening for PTSD first. However, your patient may benefit from PTSD screening at some point in the near future given its prevalence among people living unsheltered.

There are various screening tools for depression and none of them are validated specifically for the unsheltered population. For the purpose of rapid screening and commonness in primary care, this author prefers the Patient Health Questionnaire-2 (PHQ-2). Rather than use a paper questionnaire, memorize the two questions and ask them verbally. The two questions are "How often in the past two weeks have you had little interest or pleasure in doing things?" and "How often in the past two weeks have you felt down, depressed, or hopeless?" Paraphrasing the questions invalidates the screening tool and provides less useful answers. If the patient scores 3 or more, proceed with the Patient Health Questionnaire-9 (PHQ-9), which is seven additional questions after the PHQ-2. Patients who score a 10 or above on the PHQ-9 likely have depression.

Some street medicine clinicians rightly question the validity of the PHQ-9 and other questionnaires among people sleeping unsheltered, given that sleep is often disrupted, fatigue is expected, and most people imagine being homeless would naturally involve some depressed mood and anhedonia. While the PHQ-9 has not been validated in homeless populations, the Beck Depression Inventory (BDI) was found to exhibit sufficient validity and reliability among people who are homeless and precariously housed [2]. Both the BDI and the PHQ-9 contain questions about fatigue, appetite, and sleep, though these topics comprise a third of questions on the PHQ-9 compared to a fifth of the BDI. The PHQ-9 may be easier to use in the street medicine setting because it has half the number of questions and it is available in more electronic medical records.

3.12 The Value of a Diagnosis

Though the RSPA is focused on symptom clusters to inform rapid decision-making about treatment, it does not give a definitive diagnosis which you will need for documenting in the medical record and for completing forms for housing and benefits. When you document a diagnosis, pick the one that you think best fits and try to avoid "not otherwise specified" (NOS) or "undifferentiated" diagnoses. In the United States, insurance companies, the Social Security Administration, housing providers, and others do not fully understand the NOS diagnosis and often they perceive it as an "I don't really know what this is" diagnosis. They may refuse to pay for services, authorize medications, or provide benefits if your diagnosis appears uncertain. You will know that your diagnosis is a good-enough street diagnosis, but others need more certainty. Your street medicine team may not complete paperwork or assessments for social security benefits for patients, but if you believe that your patient meets criteria for disability payments (substantial impairment that has lasted 12 months or is expected to continue for another year), your diagnosis and documentation can help patients obtain benefits that can be used to obtain housing.

The diagnosis of substance-induced psychotic disorder should also be avoided if reasonable, as it can be a stigmatizing diagnosis that does not reflect the complex relationship between schizophrenia and substance use disorders. There are strong genetic links between schizophrenia and substance use disorders. As adolescent tobacco and cannabis use are associated with earlier onset of schizophrenia, they should be considered as part of the prodrome of schizophrenia rather than the cause. Other substance use disorders, such as cocaine and alcohol use disorders, are genetically linked to schizophrenia as well. Given this information, a diagnosis of substance-induced psychotic disorder may not be accurate and it is likely to make others think the psychosis would stop in the setting of abstinence. For some people the psychosis may stop, but for many others, it will not.

3.13 Assessment for ADHD

The Rapid Street Psych Assessment does not include evaluating for ADHD, though it is comorbid with many psychiatric diagnoses. Published research is mixed regarding the association between ADHD and homelessness and there is minimal research on the prevalence of ADHD within the unsheltered population. Several studies commented that ADHD appears to be associated with comorbid mental health diagnoses, but that ADHD itself is not associated with homelessness [3]. Another study cited an association between impaired impulse control and being banned from an adult homeless shelter, which suggests that people with this symptom as a part of ADHD may be at higher risk for unsheltered homelessness. Given that the Diagnostic and Statistics Manual 5th edition TR (DSM V-TR) states that ADHD is a disorder "disorder defined by impairing levels of inattention, disorganization, and/or hyperactivity-impulsivity," ADHD is likely to impair a person's ability to exit street homelessness [4].

You may want to consider completing an assessment for ADHD in a separate visit from the RSPA in order to minimize the length of any one encounter if needed. First, however, ask the person to briefly describe symptoms and when they first started, as the diagnosis of ADHD requires some symptoms to start prior to age 12. Some patients may have been diagnosed with ADHD prior to the age of 12, though you should confirm who made the diagnosis. In some children, high levels of intelligence mask symptoms both prior to and after the age of 12, confounding the ability to diagnose ADHD [5]. Additionally, privilege often dictates whether a person is diagnosed with ADHD in childhood, as ADHD diagnoses are overrepresented in white male populations [6]. If your patient's only mental health complaint is ADHD, it remains important to screen for psychosis, rule out symptoms only associated with mania, and attempt to differentiate between ADHD and symptoms that began after a childhood traumatic experience. Traumatized children often have the same symptoms as children with ADHD. Teasing apart these symptoms is challenging diagnostic work, especially when we are asking our patients to think back to childhood. Even more challenging, ADHD often presents with comorbidities, such as psychotic disorders, Bipolar disorder, Major Depressive Disorder, PTSD, and other anxiety disorders.

To aid in diagnosis, a copy of the 6-item Adult ADHD Self-report Scale Symptom Checklist (ASRS) is printed below in Fig. 3.6. Whether you use this checklist to aid in the diagnosis or have your patient complete the checklist should depend on your patient's tolerance for completing questionnaires. One benefit of the ASRS is having a baseline score to determine if a medication treatment reduces symptoms. Scoring, updated in 2024, assigns points to each response with "Never" receiving 0 points and "Very often" receiving 4 points. Scores of 14 or above are positive for ADHD.

Adult ADHD Self-Report Scale (ASRS-v1.1) Symptom Checklist

Patient Name		Today's Date				

Please answer the questions below, rating yourself on each of the criteria shown using the scale on the right side of the page. As you answer each question, place an X in the box that best describes how you have felt and conducted yourself over the past 6 months. Please give this completed checklist to your healthcare professional to discuss during today's appointment.	Never	Rarely	Sometimes	Often	Very Often
1. How often do you have trouble wrapping up the final details of a project, once the challenging parts have been done?					
2. How often do you have difficulty getting things in order when you have to do a task that requires organization?					
3. How often do you have problems remembering appointments or obligations?					
4. When you have a task that requires a lot of thought, how often do you avoid or delay getting started?					
5. How often do you fidget or squirm with your hands or feet when you have to sit down for a long time?					
6. How often do you feel overly active and compelled to do things, like you were driven by a motor?					

Fig. 3.6 Adult ADHD Self-Report Scale

3.14 Assessment for Suicidal and Homicidal Ideation

Asking about suicidal ideation (SI) and homicidal ideation (HI) is an important component of both the RSPA and every follow-up visit. Nearly one third of people who are homeless have attempted suicide during their lives [7]. Talking with patients about their suicidal and homicidal thoughts does not increase the risk a person will carry out the thoughts. Rather, it usually gives clinicians an opportunity to reduce risk. The key with each assessment is to determine the true risk associated with thoughts, as most SI and HI do not require emergency intervention. Elements to help determine level of risk include the plan for suicide or homicide, access to weapons or other means, intent, and for homicide, a target. While there are many modifiable and non-modifiable risk factors for suicide or homicide completion, these elements must be present and doable.

3.14.1 Plan

The more specific the plan for suicide or homicide, the more likely the person will accomplish the plan. A plan to commit suicide on a specific day at a specific time in a specific place with a specific weapon or means of killing oneself or others presents higher risk. A nonspecific plan, such as "I thought about killing myself today," is lower risk, especially if there is no identified means. Some people report always having a plan, such as "I could jump in front of a car or I could take an overdose." Despite these thoughts, if the person does not have a time, place, reason, weapon, or target, they are at lower risk of following through on the thoughts. One street medicine patient who was well-known by his team reported at every visit, "I'm going to kill all the politicians in Washington," but never had a time or a plan for travel, and he never named specific targets in Washington. He reported having a gun buried in the woods, but had no plan to dig it up. This person, while at some chronic elevated risk of homicide, never followed through with it during 4 years of treatment. If, however, he had developed a more detailed plan or taken any actions involved in the plan, such as digging up his gun, buying a bus ticket for Washington, D.C., intervention by the street medicine team may have been necessary.

3.14.2 Means or Weapons

Means to kill oneself or others includes weapons of any kind as well as the ability to place the person in harm's way such as jumping off a bridge or pushing someone else into traffic. When assessing risk, consider how lethal the means are and the practicality of using the means. If someone plans to take an overdose, what will they use? How much will they take? If they plan to take pills, how many milligrams are the pills? Do they already have the pills? An overdose of 30 pills of the highest dose of fluoxetine is much less lethal than an overdose of 30 pills of the lowest dose of lithium. Equally, if a patient has a knife to slice their wrists but intends to slice them across the wrist rather than lengthwise on their arms, the lethality decreases. If a person wants to use a gun to commit homicide or suicide, do they have the money for a gun or plans for how they will obtain one. Having another weapon - often people sleeping rough have a knife to protect themselves—may not increase the risk of suicide or homicide if the person has no plans to use the other weapon. Patients often specify how they want to die: "Using my knife would hurt too much. I'd rather take pills so I can die in my sleep."

3.14.3 Intent

Intent to kill oneself or others indicates elevated risk of completing the plan. A patient who says she has no reason for living, has specific lethal plans she can accomplish, and intends to kill herself would likely benefit from hospitalization, as she has a high risk of suicide completion. One method for finding wiggle room in intent to commit suicide is to gently ask, "Why haven't you done it already?". Even if she cannot identify reasons to live, she can usually find a reason she has not tried to kill herself already. Even if she cannot identify reasons to live, they can usually find a reason they have not tried to kill herself already. Fear of pain, religious consequences, or concern for the effect on a loved one are common reasons. "I really want to die, but it would kill my mother and I can't do that to her." Sometimes the response is a thoughtful "I don't know why I haven't done it yet." Oftentimes, good follow-up responses to patients expressing these thoughts uses the motivational interviewing technique of helping the person recognize that they may feel two ways about suicide or homicide. Saying, "It sounds as if on one hand, you have thought about 'X' but on the other hand you're hesitant about going through with it," can help patients recognize their conflicting thoughts and convince themselves—and you—they have less intent than they originally thought.

3.14.4 Target and Homicide Risk Factors

Identification of a target and access to the target is an essential component for homicide completion. Typically, the target is a single individual, though cases of mass shootings tend to attract more attention from the media. If your patient identifies a specific target for homicide, determine if the patient has access to the target. Patients often do not know where the person is, the person lives in a distant location, or the person is incarcerated. Despite having a specific target, lack of access to the person often impedes action. More active involvement in locating the target or traveling to where the target lives likely demonstrates increased risk. Other risk factors for homicide completion include psychotic illness, specifically with command auditory hallucinations, personality disorder diagnosis, and history of violence. Remember to evaluate your own bias when determining risk for homicide; people with mental illness and people who are homeless are both more likely to be victims of homicide than perpetrators.

3.14.5 Suicide Risk Factors

Considering risk factors will also help you determine what level of intervention you need to make. A 2023 meta-analysis, in which nearly half of participants were unsheltered, found that factors predicting SI and suicide attempt differ somewhat from factors elevating risk among housed individuals. Chronic physical illness, history of violent behavior, previous suicide attempts, previous physical abuse, mood and psychotic disorders, substance use disorders, PTSD, and personality disorders were each associated with suicide attempt. While people age of 35 and older were more likely to have previously attempted suicide, they were less likely to endorse suicidal ideation during the study period [8]. These factors are primarily chronic risk factors and do not assist in recognizing acute or imminent risk.

A PubMed search of acute risk factors for suicide attempts among homeless or unsheltered individuals produced no results. Street medicine teams working with suicidal patients will need to rely on studies of potentially dissimilar populations. A 2022 case crossover study by Bagge and colleagues assessed acute risk factors among patients hospitalized for suicide attempts, comparing emotions, cognitions, and behaviors present in the six hours prior to suicide attempt to those present during the same time one day earlier. The authors determined the following behaviors were statistically significant in the 6 hours prior to the suicide attempt: any suicide communications, any preparations for suicide, any negative interpersonal event, and any alcohol use. Feeling empty, hostile, or scared and having thoughts of being a burden and having no reason to live were also statistically significant [9]. A 2023 qualitative study further pinpointed components of suicide preparation—resolving to attempt suicide in the near future, finalizing a plan to attempt suicide, making preparations to attempt suicide and preparing personal affairs—that signaled "a dangerous shift to the individual assuming an active role in harming themselves." [10] Among people sleeping outside with few possessions, putting affairs in order may include arrangements for care of a pet.

References

1. Ayano G, Tsegay L, Abraha M, Yohannes K. Post-traumatic stress disorder among homeless people: systematic review and meta-analysis. Psychiatr Q. 2020;91(4):949–63. https://doi.org/10.1007/s11126-020-09746-1.
2. Cho LL, Jones AA, Barbic S, Leonova O, Vila-Rodriguez F, Buchanan T, et al. Psychometric properties and correlates of the Beck Depression Inventory in a community-based and homeless or precariously housed sample. J Affect Disord Rep. 2021;6:100229. https://doi.org/10.1016/j.jadr.2021.100229.
3. Riglin L, Todd A, Blakey R, Shakeshaft A, Stergiakouli E, Davey Smith G, et al. Investigating young-adult social outcomes of attention deficit hyperactivity disorder. J Clin Psychiatry. 2023;84(2):22m14379. https://doi.org/10.4088/JCP.22m14379.
4. Koutsoklenis A, Honkasilta J. ADHD in the DSM-5-TR: what has changed and what has not. Front Psychiatry. 2023;13:1064141. https://doi.org/10.3389/fpsyt.2022.1064141.
5. Cadenas M, Hartman CA, Faraone SV, Antshel KM, Borges Á, Hoogeveen L, et al. Cognitive correlates of attention-deficit hyperactivity disorder in children and adolescents with high intellectual ability. J Neurodev Disord. 2020;12(1):7. https://doi.org/10.1186/s11689-020-9307-8.
6. Shalaby N, Sengupta S, Williams JB. Large-scale analysis reveals racial disparities in the prevalence of ADHD and conduct disorders. Sci Rep. 2024;14(1):75954. https://doi.org/10.1038/s41598-024-75954-5.
7. Xiang J, Kaminga AC, Wu XY, Lai Z, Yang J, Lian Y, et al. Lifetime prevalence of suicidal attempt among homeless individuals in North America: a meta-analysis. J Affect Disord. 2021;294:145–53. https://doi.org/10.1016/j.jad.2021.07.066.
8. Armoon B, Griffiths MD, Mohammadi R, Ahounbar E. Suicidal behaviors and risk taking among homeless individuals: a systematic review and meta-analysis. Commun Ment Health J. 2023;59(7):1283–99. https://doi.org/10.1007/s10597-023-01111-3.
9. Bagge CL, Littlefield AK, Wiegand TJ, Hawkins E, Trim RS, Schumacher JA, et al. A controlled examination of acute warning signs for suicide attempts among hospitalized patients. J Clin Psychiatry. 2023;84(2):22m14606. https://doi.org/10.4088/JCP.22m14606.
10. Conner KR, Kearns JC, Denneson LM. Qualitative analysis of hospital patient narratives of warning signs on the day of their suicide attempt. J Affect Disord. 2023;326:329–35. https://doi.org/10.1016/j.jad.2023.01.080.

Medication Treatment of Mental Disorders

4

4.1 Introduction

This chapter offers information to equip clinicians to safely prescribe psychotropic medications to people living unsheltered if they consent to taking medications. The medications discussed are used within the United States (U.S.) and listed by their generic name with the U.S. brand name in parentheses. Brand names are included solely for readers who are not familiar with generic medication names. Generic medications, where available, are preferred because of cost. While all of the medications in this chapter are approved by the U.S. Food and Drug Administration (FDA), pharmaceutical companies have not sought FDA approval for each medication in a class for every diagnosis the class can treat. For this reason, psychiatrists routinely prescribe medications off-label.

4.2 Consent for Treatment

Building trust during all interactions with your patient is the most important component of street medicine work and cannot be emphasized enough. While this chapter discusses the appropriate medications to prescribe based on symptom cluster with specific considerations for the street environment, the decision to participate in medication treatment *always* remains with the person living on the streets. As stated in Chap. 3, I start all discussions about medications by telling the patient, "If you decide to try a medication and you hate how it makes you feel, just stop taking it. I will never make you continue a medication you hate. It's your body and you get to decide what goes in it."

With regard to ability to consent, people who have psychotic or other mental health symptoms are capable of consenting for treatment and making informed decisions. The patient does need to be able to understand the potential benefits and the potential side effects of a medication and agree to take the medication. Following the harm-reduction approach to prescribing mitigates risk and reduces

S. Hatcher et al., *Street Mental Health Handbook*,
https://doi.org/10.1007/978-3-032-00663-9_4

the level of cognition required to consent. Sometimes a capacity evaluation may need to be performed in order to determine if the person can consent to a specific treatment/procedure or to determine if they lack capacity to refuse something potentially life-saving. See Chap. 7, Sect. 7.4 for information on capacity assessments. In the United States, medications typically cannot be administered if the person refuses the medication, with exceptions for life-endangering situations and court order. States vary in laws regarding involuntary treatment on inpatient psychiatric units and in certain circumstances, if two physicians agree, medication treatment can be forced. Attempting to force medication on the streets is not only impractical but also traumatizing and highly likely to result in disengagement from treatment.

Most organizations within the United States require patients to sign a consent-to-treat form. Many street medicine teams work under the umbrella of clinics or health systems, and consents used for treating patients indoors are sufficient for street medicine. Many acceptable consent-to-treat examples can be found online if needed. Some patients may only be willing to provide verbal consent, particularly in the setting of paranoia. When a patient provides verbal consent only, document it in the medical record.

4.3 A Harm Reduction Approach to Prescribing

Many psychiatric diagnoses impair cognition, reduce energy and motivation, and cause high levels of anxiety or paranoia when interacting with others. A person experiencing these symptoms will likely have difficulty navigating tasks required to secure housing, even in locations that provide low barrier access to housing. Prescribers should consider which is more harmful, continued exposure to the harms of the streets or medication side effects and adverse effects. The harm-reduction approach to prescribing helps clinicians consider the myriad potential harms involved in treating and not treating the health conditions of someone sleeping rough. Harms of the street include exposure to physical and sexual violence, the weather, pollution, stigma, and other traumas, which are often not considered by clinicians hesitant to prescribe psychiatric medications in the street medicine setting. Figure 4.1 below demonstrates the harms clinicians must weigh when considering a specific medication for someone sleeping rough. In each class of psychotropic medications, there are medication options in which the benefits outweigh the risks and can substantially improve mental health among street medicine patients.

Table 4.1 below lists risks and benefits of medications to consider for psychotropic medications. While there are risks for many medications, none are absolutely contraindicated on the streets. Because local communities and street medicine teams have different attributes and resources, one medication may be unsafe in one set of conditions yet safe in another. As new medications come to market after the publication of this handbook, these risks and benefits can help determine which medications you can safely prescribe on the streets.

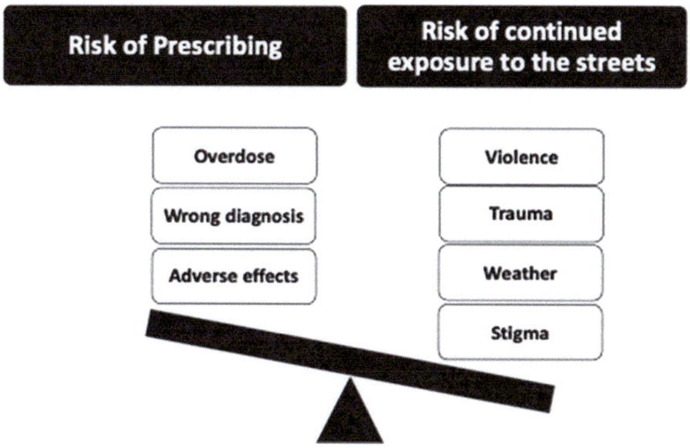

Fig. 4.1 Comparison of the Harms of Medications and Remaining Unsheltered

Table 4.1 Medication risks to consider when prescribing

Risk	Medications
Victimization from over-sedation	Quetiapine, risperidone, paliperidone, olanzapine, trazodone, diphenhydramine, ziprasidone
Adverse effects from missed doses	Venlafaxine, paroxetine, lamotrigine, clozapine
Overdose risk	Tricyclic antidepressants (e.g. amitriptyline), lithium, valproic acid
Poor absorption due to poor access to food	Ziprasidone, lurasidone
Difficulty monitoring adverse effects	EKG—Ziprasidone, haloperidol, tricyclic antidepressants; Blood draws—lithium, valproic acid, carbamazepine, clozapine
Misuse or diversion potential	Benzodiazepines, quetiapine, bupropion, clonidine, gabapentin, buprenorphine, stimulants to treat ADHD
Fetal anomalies during pregnancy	Lithium, valproic acid, lamotrigine
Refrigeration needed	Injectable formulations of naltrexone, buprenorphine, risperidone
Problematic with dehydration	Lithium

4.4 Genetic Testing

The evidence for genetic testing is mixed and routine genetic testing is not recommended at this time. The tests identify genetic variations that control how fast the liver metabolizes certain medications, unlike genetic ancestry tests. As the science evolves, genetic tests may prove more useful. In the street medicine setting, genetic testing can be helpful in several scenarios. The typical method for finding the right medication is trial and error and avoidance of certain side effects. By the time people with mental health diagnoses end up on the streets, they have often tried a pharmacopeia of psychotropic medications. Genetic testing can help shorten the list of medications to trial. Genetic testing helps some patients feel more comfortable with taking medications, particularly in the setting of Obsessive Compulsive Disorder (OCD) where patients can become paralyzed by "what if" scenarios. Last, genetic testing can help identify reasons some patients have not done well on numerous medications, as there are some genetic variations that cause people to metabolize medications in unexpected ways. Be cautious when offering genetic testing to patients with psychotic disorders who experience a high burden of paranoia. Some may suspect you have nefarious motives for wanting to collect their genetic information.

4.5 Antipsychotics

If you determine that a patient has either bipolar disorder (with or without psychotic symptoms) or psychosis (regardless of the diagnosis), prescribe an antipsychotic. See Sect. 4.6 on mood stabilizing medication for an explanation of why antipsychotics are better suited for bipolar disorder within street medicine. The treatment goal with antipsychotics on the streets is to improve functioning in order to accomplish tasks required to move into housing. Though some people may achieve symptom remission while sleeping outside, the chaotic environment of the streets makes remission challenging. Even if housing is readily available, there is no need to wait to move someone into housing to start treating symptoms; transition into housing is rarely a straight smooth path.

4.5.1 Antipsychotic Selection and Prescribing

There are many antipsychotics from which to choose. Select an antipsychotic that has worked well for the person in the past, as long as there are not any major safety issues for someone sleeping rough. If the patient does not have a preference or is antipsychotic-naïve, select the medication based on its risk profile and/or its availability as a long-acting injectable. See the antipsychotic selection decision tree in Fig. 4.2 below for help identifying the best first choice antipsychotic.

Aripiprazole (Abilify) is not sedating and has a lower risk profile on the streets, it is a good first choice and is available in a LAI formulation. Though oral risperidone (Risperdal) and paliperidone (Invega) are sedating, they are also available in long-acting injectable formulations that are not sedating. For patients who have daily access to one caloric meal per day, lurasidone is a nonsedating oral option, but it does not have a LAI formulation. Many individuals living unsheltered eat only a few meals per week and survive the rest of the time on snacks, which may not meet the 350+ calorie requirement for lurasidone. Quetiapine (Seroquel) and olanzapine (Zyprexa) are effective antipsychotics, but can be too sedating for many people sleeping outside to tolerate given safety concerns. Olanzapine is particularly known for causing rapid weight gain, though all antipsychotics have that capacity, and weight should be checked regularly if it is prescribed. Weight gain may be mitigated among people sleeping rough because they walk a lot. Once patients move indoors, however, the weight gain can be profound. Quetiapine does have a street value and may need to be avoided for that reason. Most patients tell me it is valuable for avoiding withdrawal effects from crack/cocaine. Given that withdrawal from cocaine can

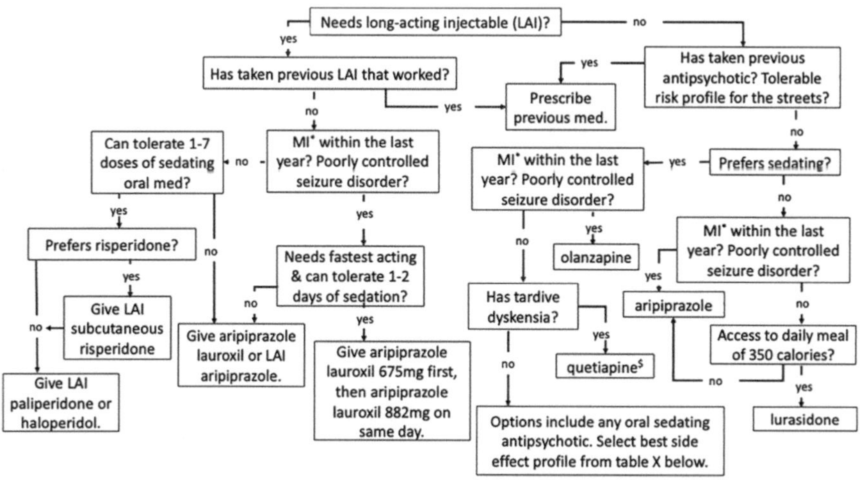

Fig. 4.2 Antipsychotic selection decision tree. *Myocardial infarction. $Only prescribe quetiapine if diversion risk is low in your local area. Otherwise, select olanzapine and/or treat tardive dyskinesia separately

cause irritability and suicidal ideation, I do not consider this to be the worst street use of an antipsychotic. However, if your patients sell their quetiapine instead of taking it for the intended use, it obviously won't improve their symptoms.

Drug interactions are common between psychiatric medications and with medications for other health problems. Avoid combining more than one antipsychotic for people sleeping outside. If a patient has taken a combination of antipsychotics in the past, just start with one medication. Generally, antipsychotics and antidepressants can be safely prescribed in combination, though many electronic health records will show a medication interaction. Some of the warnings include QTc prolongation and risk of serotonin syndrome. There is a small risk for serotonin syndrome, but the risk can be minimized by prescribing no more than two agents that increase the risk. Avoid ziprasidone and escitalopram/citalopram combinations if concerned for QTc prolongation risk. Use a drug interaction checker either online or through your electronic health record when selecting an antipsychotic.

4.5.1.1 Oral Antipsychotics

Many oral antipsychotic medications are available on the market and can be prescribed inexpensively. In Table 4.2 below, the asterisk indicates oral antipsychotics that are available in the United States as a generic medication. Some psychiatric inpatient units prescribe medications without thoughtfulness about the cost to the patient upon discharge. You may need to switch oral antipsychotics to provide one that is covered by the patient's insurance or is sufficiently inexpensive to include on your street medicine formulary.

Below, Table 4.2 provides information on dosing for many antipsychotics available in the United States and Canada, though you may not want to use all of them in

Table 4.2 Oral antipsychotic medication dosing

Medication	Starting dose	Next dose	Next dose	Next dose	Max dose	Other
Aripiprazole (Abilify)	5 mg	10 mg	15 mg	20 mg	30 mg	Can increase by 5–10 mg
Asenapine (Saphris)	5–10 mg	10 mg	20 mg	–	20 mg	Sublingual
Brexipiprazole (Rexulti)	1 mg on days 1–4	2 mg on days 5–7	4 mg	–	4mg	
Cariprazine (Vraylar)	1.5 mg on day 1	3 mg on day 2	Increase by 1.5 to 3 mg increments up to max		6 mg	
Clozapine (Clozaril)	25 mg	50 mg	100 mg	150 mg	400+ mg	Check absolute neutrophil count weekly to every other week. Titrate to 200 mg by the end of week 2
Fluphenazine (Prolixin)	0.5 mg TID—QID	1 mg TID—QID	1.5 mg TID—QID	2 mg TID—QID	10 mg TID—QID	Maintenance doses of 3 mg or more are rarely needed. If the dose is titrated higher in the initial phase of symptom control, try to slowly reduce the dose lower than 3 mg/day. Maintenance doses can be given once daily
Haloperidol (Haldol)	2–5 mg	5 mg	10 mg	15mg	40 mg	Most psychiatrists use no more than 20 mg per day
Iloperidone (Fanapt)	2 mg	4 mg	6 mg	12 mg	24 mg	Look up dosing instructions to titrate slowly over 1–2 weeks. Must start over if off med for 4+ days
Lumateperone (Calypta)	42 mg	–	–	–	42mg	No titration needed
Lurasidone (Latuda)	20–40 mg	40 mg	60 mg	80 mg	120 mg	Take with 350+ calories of food

(continued)

Table 4.2 (continued)

Medication	Starting dose	Next dose	Next dose	Next dose	Max dose	Other
Olanzapine (Zyprexa)	5–10 mg	10 mg	15 or 20 mg	30 mg	40 mg	
Paliperidone (Invega)	3 mg	6 mg	9 mg	12 mg	12 mg	
Quetiapine (Seroquel)	100–200 mg	200 mg	400 mg	600 mg	800 mg	
Risperidone (Risperdal)	1–2 mg	2 mg	4 mg	8 mg	8 mg	
Ziprasidone (Geodon)	20–40 mg	80 mg	160 mg	220 mg	220 mg	Take with 500 calories of food
Xanomeline/ Tros-pium (Cobenfy)	Two 50/20 mg capsules	Two 100/20 mg capsules	Two 125/30 mg capsules	–	250/60 mg	

the street medicine setting. Psychiatrists usually give lower starting doses to people who have never taken antipsychotics before, may be particularly sensitive to side effects, or have severe liver/kidney disease. Specific dosing instructions for patients with liver and kidney disease can be found online. Many antipsychotics are supposed to be prescribed twice daily (BID). On the streets, however, BID dosing can be difficult for patients to remember and will cause daytime sedation for most medications. On the streets, dose the total amount at bedtime or whenever the patient prefers to sleep. Because medications affect different people differently, some patients may have insomnia with a bedtime dosing, in which case, have the patient switch to morning dosing.

With a few exceptions, medications in Table 4.2 are effective only at their midrange and higher doses. For example, quetiapine 200 mg is not typically a sufficient antipsychotic dose for patients with schizophrenia or schizoaffective disorder. Lumateperone does not require titration and is considered effective at its only dose of 42 mg. Cariprazine may be effective at its lowest dose of 1.5 mg, whereas some patients will not have sufficient symptom relief until titrating to 6 mg. When a medication is ineffective at a lower dose, psychiatrists generally increase to the highest dose before switching, as long as the patient finds side effects minimal and/or tolerable. Avoid prescribing more than one antipsychotic at a time unless cross titrating.

Most medications in Table 4.2, except where indicated, can be titrated over the course of a week if necessary. Often, however, titration over the course of two or more weeks may be necessary depending on the frequency your team sees the person. Because of the cognitive impairment patients experience due to psychosis, substance use, and the chaos of the streets, titration between visits can prove difficult. For this reason, you may opt to start a higher dose of a tablet and tell the person to break it in half for the first 3–4 days, then take the whole pill. Obviously for capsules and sublingual medications, halving the dose is not possible and you may choose not to include medications in your formulary.

Before prescribing clozapine and iloperidone, carefully consider the risks and benefits. Both medications must be increased slowly over the course of 1 to 2 weeks to avoid adverse effects. They can both cause orthostatic hypotension and a fast clozapine titration is associated with higher risk of myocarditis. Equally, if a patient misses more than 3 days of these medications, the lowest dose must be restarted and the same slow titration should follow. Of the two, clozapine has a much higher benefit–risk ratio. Street psychiatry teams that prescribe clozapine often start the patient first on a long-acting injectable antipsychotic such as paliperidone palmitate to improve cognition and ability to adhere to the requirements of clozapine titration and maintenance.

4.5.1.2 Long-Acting Injectable Antipsychotics

Some oral antipsychotics are available as long-acting injectables (LAI). Most street medicine teams prefer long-acting injectables for a variety of reasons. For one, patients only need to choose to take their medication once or twice per month, rather than daily, increasing the likelihood that the patient receives a consistent effective medication level. Unlike oral medications, injectables cannot be lost or stolen, or trashed during an encampment sweep. Though patients can be reluctant to take a LAI at first, many eventually prefer one, especially if they are tired of losing or having medications stolen. Others prefer the LAI because it largely will not sedate them.

If you can find evidence, either in the medical record or in the records of a local hospital, that the patient has ever taken an oral formulation of the long-acting injectable, you can initiate the long-acting injectable without giving oral tablets first. Whether you prefer to have documentation of the person taking the oral formulation or rely on patient report depends on your comfort level. If the patient has never taken the oral medication, give at least one oral dose to avoid the risk of an allergic or dystonic reaction to a LAI that will stay in the body for two weeks or longer. Because paliperidone is the active metabolite of risperidone, prior history with oral risperidone or oral paliperidone is sufficient prior to giving the LAI paliperidone palmitate and LAI formulations of risperidone. If possible, watch the patient take the first oral dose and give additional pills to last until the next visit when you will give the LAI. If the patient only takes the first pill, you can still give the LAI; if they take the other pills, consider it icing on the cake. Most dystonic reactions occur within 5 days of giving a medication, with 50% occurring in the first 48 h [1].

Though there are numerous information documents for long-acting injectable antipsychotics, Table 4.3 combines information most useful for the streets. If you are interested in additional information, see the package insert or search for LAI reference guides. In the United States, Medicaid often pays for LAIs without prior authorization for indications of schizophrenia and schizoaffective disorder [2]. You will need to select one of these diagnoses when prescribing a LAI in order for it to be approved. Most patients with private insurance in the U.S. can access co-pay assistance cards and patients without insurance may need to rely on samples. In countries with universal health care coverage or a national health service, there may be limitations on the LAI you can select for cost-containment reasons.

Characteristics of several LAI antipsychotics limit their practicality for street medicine. Both formulations of risperidone microspheres (Risperdal Consta and Rykindo) have to be refrigerated and have only 7 days they can be kept out of the refrigerator. They, along with fluphenazine decanoate and olanzapine, are dosed every two weeks, making them less ideal than medications dosed monthly or longer. The only LAI not included in Table 4.3 is long-acting olanzapine (Zyprexa Relprevv). Due to the possibility of post-injection delirium, patients taking long-acting olanzapine need to be observed for 3 h.

Table 4.3 Long-acting Injectable Antipsychotic Dosing [3–6]

Medication	Dosing	Oral equivalent	Oral supplement	What to do for missed doses
Aripiprazole (Abilify Maintena)	400 mg or 300 mg Q4 weeks IM (300 mg dose is for slow CYP2D6 metabolizers)	15 mg	Yes, for 2 weeks with 15 mg daily	Give next dose of 400 mg as soon as possible after missed monthly injection
Aripiprazole lauroxil (Aristada)	Give 882 mg IM on day 1 and Q 28 days if psychosis persists. Try lowering the dose in subsequent months or extend for less frequent dosing if tolerated	20 mg daily: 882 mg Q4weeks; 15 mg daily: 882 mg Q6 weeks or 1064 mg Q8 weeks or 662 mg Q4 weeks; 10 mg daily: 441 mg Q 4 weeks	Combine 882 mg with aripiprazole lauroxil 675 mg and a single 30 mg oral dose on day 1 to avoid oral	Administer next injection as soon as possible. Oral supplementation or 675 mg IM may be required depending on dose strength and date of last dose
Aripiprazole lauroxil 675 mg (Aristada Initio)	Inject on day 1 with first monthly aripiprazole lauroxil dose (882mg) IM	Not applicable	Give 30 mg oral once to take on day 1 with monthly 882 mg and 675 mg doses	Not applicable; single time use when starting monthly aripiprazole lauroxil without 3 weeks of oral supplementation
Fluphenazine decanoate (Prolixin decanoate)	If on a consistent oral dose, multiply by 1.25 mg for initial dose. Otherwise, Inject 25 mg IM on day 1, then 25 mg IM Q 2 weeks. May increase by 25 mg Q 2 weeks	Oral dose multiplied by 1.25	Yes, for 3–5 weeks ideally	If missed dose is within 4 weeks of day 1, give 25 mg IM ASAP and give oral doses if patient has psychotic symptoms. If missed dose is after steady state (>4–6 weeks from initial dose), give missed dose ASAP. If 24+ weeks after last injection, give 25 mg IM and supplement with oral med for 3–5 weeks*

(continued)

Table 4.3 (continued)

Medication	Dosing	Oral equivalent	Oral supplement	What to do for missed doses
Haloperidol decanoate (Haldol decanoate)	Day 1: 50 mg IM if not consistently taking oral tablets or 100 mg IM if adherent to oral tablets. Give an additional 50 mg IM between days 4–8 if initial dose was 50 mg. Monthly injections of total dose given Q4 weeks from 2nd initial injection. Increase by 50 mg at each monthly injection if psychotic symptoms are not improved	IM dose divided by 10 (150 mg IM = 15 mg PO)	Yes, at least 6 weeks. May taper oral if EPS or other side effects occur	If steady state not reached (<3 months of therapy), give last IM dose ASAP and supplement with oral if psychosis recurs. If steady state reached, (3+ months of therapy), give last dose used ASAP. If 13+ weeks since last dose, restart initiation
Paliperidone palmitate (Invega Sustenna)	Give 234 mg IM on day 1 and 156 mg IM 4–7 days later. Monthly doses of 117 mg, 156 mg, and 234 mg are available. Give lower doses if side effects are prominent and higher doses if psychotic symptoms are not improved after the first 2 loading doses	3 mg po daily = 39–78 mg IM 6 mg po daily = 117 mg IM	None	See package insert for detailed instructions on management after a missed initiation dose and missed monthly dose
Risperidone microspheres (Risperdal Consta)[a]	25 mg IM Q2w. Increase by 12.5 mg every 4 weeks up to a max dose of 50 mg IM Q2 weeks		Yes, for 21 days	Administer missed dose ASAP. If patient reached steady state (>2 months of therapy) and missed dose was no more than 6 weeks ago, no oral doses needed. If not at steady state or >6 weeks since last injection, supplement with oral for 21 days

(continued)

Table 4.3 (continued)

Medication	Dosing	Oral equivalent	Oral supplement	What to do for missed doses
Risperidone microspheres (Rykindo)[a]	Give 25 mg IM on day 1 and on day 14. Dosed Q2w. May increase by 12.5 mg every 4 weeks. Max dose is 50 mg IM Q2w. Gluteal IM only	No oral dose equivalent listed	Yes, 7 days	Package insert reports that there is no data for missed injections, but recommends to restart at the dose last missed if the patient's general medical condition is unchanged. Supplement with oral for 7 days
Risperidone, subcutaneous (Uzedy)[b]	Package insert recommends switching once established on oral dose. If starting from 2 mg oral equivalent, considering increasing SQ dose Q4 weeks. Inject SQ into back of upper arm or abdomen	Every 50 mg SQ Q4w or 100 mg SQ Q8w equals 2 mg PO daily. Max dose 125 mg SQ Q4w or 250 mg SQ Q8w	Discontinue oral immediately	Package insert recommends to give the missed dose as soon as possible and does not comment on when to reinitiate

[a]Requires refrigeration and cannot be left out of the refrigerator for >7 days. See package insert for specific refrigeration requirements. Not recommended for most street medicine patients
[b]Requires refrigeration, but can be kept out of the refrigerator for up to 90 days if you cannot find the patient on street rounds

Recommendations for continuing oral medications during the first few weeks after initiation of some LAIs, though ideal, can be challenging for some rough sleepers. Without the oral supplement, an adequate level of LAI will eventually build up in the body to provide sufficient antipsychotic effect.

4.5.2 Antipsychotic Side Effects and Their Management

While side effects listed in this section may appear daunting, they remain important tools for street medicine teams to improve the debilitating effects of psychosis and bipolar disorder. Rather than intending to frighten you away from prescribing antipsychotics, this chapter aims to provide you with the knowledge you need to safely manage antipsychotic treatment given the dearth of mental health professionals working in street medicine. Additionally, patients benefit when all team members can recognize and report side effects to the team's prescriber. Table 4.4 below compares antipsychotics based on side effects.

Table 4.4 Antipsychotic side effect comparisons [7–12]

Medication	Sedation	Weight gain	Extra-pyramidal symptoms	Elevated prolactin	QTc risk	Seizure risk
Aripiprazole (Abilify)	+	+	+	–	–	+
Asenapine (Saphris)	++	++	+	+	++	+?
Brexipiprazole (Rexulti)	+	+	–	–	–	+?
Cariprazine (Vraylar)	+	+	+	–	–	+?
Chlorpromazine (Thorazine)	+++	+++	++	++	+++	+++
Clozapine (Clozaril)	+++	+++	—	—	++	+++
Fluphenazine (Prolixin)	–	+	+++	+++	+++	++
Haloperidol (Haldol)	++	+	+++	+++	+	++
Iloperidone (Fanapt)	++	+++	–	+	++	+?
Lumateperone (Calypta)	++	–	–	–	–	+?
Lurasidone (Latuda)	+	+	+	++	—	+?
Olanzapine (Zyprexa)	+++	+++	+/–	+	+	++
Paliperidone (Invega)	++	++	++	+++	+	+/–
Quetiapine (Seroquel)	+++	+++	–	–	+	++
Risperidone (Risperdal)	++	++	++	+++	+	++
Ziprasidone (Geodon)	+++	–	++	+	+++	+
Xanomeline/Trospium (Cobenfy)	–	–	–	–	–	–

– – opposite effect; – minimal/no effect; + mild effect; ++ moderate effect; +++ marked effect; +/– evidence is mixed; +? insufficient evidence for comparison but package insert indicates risk

4.5.2.1 Sedation

Few antipsychotics do not cause sedation; aripiprazole, brexipiprazole, cariprazine, lumateperone, haloperidol, lurasidone, and fluphenazine are the least sedating of options and may be preferred by patients. As described in this chapter's section on harm reduction prescribing, remember to have a careful conversation with your patients related to sedation from antipsychotics. Long-acting injectable antipsychotics tend not to sedate patients on an ongoing basis, though some can cause sedation within the first several days of initiation.

4.5.2.2 Metabolic Effects

Weight gain, dyslipidemia, and elevated blood glucose are common side effects of antipsychotics. Even those advertised to be more metabolically neutral are not benign. Some may cause less weight gain but more problems with blood glucose or lipids. Olanzapine and clozapine are associated with the highest weight gain [13]. Lower starting BMI and weight gain of 5% of body weight in the first month are both associated with longer-term weight gain [14]. Numerous factors pose challenges in monitoring these side effects among unsheltered individuals: inability to evaluate fasting labs, difficulty obtaining any labs, access to point-of-care hemoglobin A1c machines, multiple layers of clothing limiting evaluation of waist circumference, and inaccurate weights from using a scale on uneven ground to name a few. While overweight and obesity are problematic within the homeless population, they are less common among unsheltered individuals due to higher levels of physical activity such as walking to access services and poor access to food [15–17]. Equally, inconsistent medication adherence, which is expected in the street medicine setting, may also minimize the metabolic impacts of antipsychotics.

Switching to a less offending antipsychotic, lifestyle changes, and metformin are the predominant recommended interventions for both preventing and treating antipsychotic-induced weight gain and, when implemented before a gain of 7% of body weight, these interventions are most helpful among people with psychotic disorders [18]. Recommending lifestyle changes to someone sleeping outside can cause them to disengage with you, as they have such little control over their food options and ability to engage in formal exercise. Metformin is the best option for mitigating metabolic side effects if the patient needs to remain on the antipsychotic causing weight gain. The extended release formulation can limit gastrointestinal side effects and offers preferred once daily dosing. That said, less is more with regard to medication regimens in the street medicine setting. Pill burden and cognitive impairments pose risks related to confusion about one's medication regimen and discontinuation. If the patient starts a long-acting antipsychotic or when they are able to move into housing, monitor metabolic side effects more closely as adherence improves with LAIs and physical activity tends to decline with moving indoors.

4.5.2.3 Extrapyramidal Signs (EPS)

EPS vary from nearly imperceptible, such as a mild tremor, to very impairing and disfiguring full body involuntary movement and are neurologic effects of antipsychotic medications. Types of EPS include dystonia, akathisia, tardive dyskinesia, parkinsonism, catatonia, and neuroleptic malignant syndrome (NMS). Use of cocaine, methamphetamine, ecstasy, and bath salts (synthetic cathinones) can cause EPS in the absence of an antipsychotic and increase the risk and severity of EPS when used concomitantly with an antipsychotic [19–21]. All antipsychotics can cause EPS and some have low risk for one type and high risk for another type. Treatment of EPS can be found in Table 4.5.

The standard measure of evaluating abnormal movements is the Abnormal Involuntary Movement Scale (AIMS) which is public domain and available online. The AIMS requires the patient to engage in some interesting movements, which may be embarrassing to perform on the street in front of others. Even in a private clinic room, patients find the AIMS bizarre. Performing the test with the patient demonstrates how to perform its components and may improve their willingness to participate. There are some extremely boring YouTube videos that teach you how to use the AIMS, as well as recognize and assess involuntary movements. These videos are helpful to watch if you are not a psychiatrist or do not have experience recognizing abnormal movements.

Acute Dystonia Described as sustained, slow, twisting, painful muscle spasms that can cause abnormal postures, acute dystonia typically starts within hours to a few days

Table 4.5 Outpatient medication management for EPS

Medication	Indication	Starting dose	Next dose	Typical max street dose	Other
Benztropine (Cogentin)	TD, akathisia, dystonia	1 mg Qhs	2 mg Qhs	2mg BID	Sedating
Deutetrabenazine (Austedo)	TD	6 mg BID	9 mg BID	48 mg BID	Check QTc before dosing above 24 mg in at risk patients. Must re-titrate if stopped for >1 week
Diphenhydramine (Benadryl)	TD, akathisia, dystonia	25 mg Qhs	50 mg Qhs	100 mg Qhs (can divide BID)	Sedating
Propranolol (Inderal)	Akathisia	10 mg Qhs	20 mg Qhs	40 mg Qhs or divided BID	Lowers blood pressure
Mirtazapine (Remeron)	Akathisia	7.5 mg Qhs	15 mg Qhs	15 mg Qhs for akathisia	Sedating
Valbenazine (Ingrezza)	TD	40 mg Qam	80 mg Qam	80 mg Qam	May increase to 80 mg daily after 1 week of initial dose
Vitamin B6	Akathisia	600 mg Qam	None	600 mg Qam	

after initiation of an antipsychotic and occur in roughly 2–5% of patients. Dystonia can be generalized involving the trunk and other motor groups or, most commonly, restricted to the head, neck, mouth, jaw, and eyes [22]. Risperidone, haloperidol, fluphenazine, and other high-potency first generation antipsychotics most commonly cause dystonia. Other risk factors include younger age, male sex, substance use, and previous dystonia [23]. Clozapine and quetiapine cause dystonia at the same rate as placebo. Cessation of the antipsychotic typically resolves the dystonia within 48 h [24]. Treatment in an emergency room is strongly encouraged and necessary if the dystonia involves airway restriction or difficulty swallowing. Treatment includes anticholinergic, antihistamine, or benzodiazepine treatment. Intramuscular treatment is more effective than oral medication and intravenous medication should be used if the airway is compromised. Because acute dystonic reactions can cause mistrust among patients, some prescribers prefer to give a prophylactic anticholinergic medication. Amantadine (Symmetrel) 100 mg one to three times daily can be used as an alternative to anticholinergics and can produce insomnia, which some patients may prefer over a sedating prophylactic [25]. For a variety of reasons, you may choose to reserve prophylaxis for patients at high risk in the street medicine setting.

Akathisia Akathisia, chronically underrecognized, is a side effect of antipsychotic medications described by an intense inner restlessness and need to move constantly. It is often confused with anxiety and agitation, which can result from akathisia. Often presenting in the lower limbs, ranging from shaking or tapping feet to pacing, patients can briefly and uncomfortably control the movements. Akathisia has been associated with suicidal ideation among some patients, though research is mixed [26]. Acute onset occurs within a few days to a few weeks with starting an antipsychotic and rapid titration, particularly with lurasidone, lumateperone, haloperidol, and cariprazine [27]. Withdrawal akathisia occurs within two weeks of discontinuing some antipsychotics and can last up to six weeks.

Similar to dystonia, akathisia can drive a wedge between patients and prescribers. In this author's experience, patients often stop the antipsychotic immediately, particularly in severe cases, and refuse other antipsychotics. Whether the akathisia is caused by an antipsychotic or withdrawal of an antipsychotic, treatment is effective. Mirtazapine 7.5 to 15 mg nightly and Vitamin B6 600 mg daily have the best efficacy for akathisia with vitamin B6 more useful for street medicine due to lack of sedation [28]. Other treatments include GABA agonists and modulators such as benzodiazepines, pregabalin (Lyrica), and gabapentin (Neurontin); dopamine agonists such as amantadine (Symmetrel), and antihistamines such as diphenhydramine (Benadryl), and propranolol. None of these medications are without risk in the street medicine setting; weighing the risks and benefits for each patient and within your local medication misuse context is important.

Tardive Dyskinesia (TD) TD is a side effect of antipsychotics, but can also be caused by some substances such as methamphetamine, cocaine, and bath salts. It is characterized by involuntary, repetitive, and uncontrollable or briefly controllable movements that start typically months or years after medication is initiated. Movements may be choreiform in nature. Older age, female sex, first generation antipsychotics, higher doses, and lengthy periods of antipsychotic treatment are all risk factors for TD. Without intervention, TD usually worsens in severity of movements and parts of the body affected. TD may persist for years past cessation of all medications and substances. Patients may be aware and distressed by the movements or unaware of their existence.

When considering treatment for TD, first try lowering the dose if the patient is not having ongoing psychotic symptoms. Next, switch to an antipsychotic less likely to cause TD, such as quetiapine or clozapine if possible within your street medicine setting. If the person needs to remain on an antipsychotic that worsens or causes TD and cannot tolerate a dose change, add a medication to treat the side effect. As with all patients, prescribing as few medications as possible is preferable and is particularly important for people with cognitive impairment. See Table E below for treatments of EPS. Research is mixed regarding whether anticholinergic medications such as benztropine and diphenhydramine improve or worsen tardive dyskinesia, though they have been used to treat the disorder for many years. Pramipexole, a dopamine agonist, is an alternative to anticholinergics that can relieve dyskinesia symptoms, but may worsen psychosis. Benzodiazepines can also improve TD symptoms, though the risks likely do not outweigh the benefits in the street medicine setting.

Parkinsonism Parkinsonism, more common with older age, first-generation antipsychotics, higher antipsychotic dose, and female sex, presents similarly to Parkinson's disease and can be difficult to distinguish. Some readers may remember the "Thorazine shuffle" common in the days prior to second-generation antipsychotics, as up to 50% of patients taking chlorpromazine (Thorazine) develop parkinsonism. Risperidone, paliperidone, and olanzapine have higher risk among second-generation antipsychotics, whereas clozapine and quetiapine have low to no risk. Parkinsonism is typically described as asymmetric with bradykinesia (slowed movements) and rigidity being the most prominent symptoms. Don't be fooled, however, by tremor at rest, shuffling gait, and symmetry, as half of antipsychotic-induced parkinsonism cases present this way. Strategies for people with psychotic disorders include lowering the antipsychotic dose or switching to an antipsychotic less associated with parkinsonism. These strategies are also preferred in the street medicine setting, as opposed to adding a medication to treat parkinsonism. Treatment with anticholinergics, such as benztropine (Cogentin) and trihexyphenidyl (Artane), is common but less safe among older adults and people sleeping unsheltered. While amantadine (Symmetrel) may be a safer alternative, watch for increased psychosis.

Neuroleptic Malignant Syndrome (NMS) NMS is a rare, but potentially life threatening adverse reaction to antipsychotics. Characterized by lead-pipe rigidity, fever, altered mental status, and autonomic dysfunction (wild swings in blood pressure, rapid pulse, sweating), NMS should be treated in the hospital [29]. Though it has some overlapping symptoms with serotonin syndrome (discussed later in this chapter with side effects of antidepressants), NMS is more common with first-generation antipsychotics. Serotonin syndrome is more likely to occur with second-generation antipsychotics and usually in combination with other serotonergic agents [30]. Other distinguishing features include reduced bowel sounds, bradykinesia, and cogwheel rigidity with NMS compared to serotonin syndrome. While muscle rigidity can occur with serotonin syndrome, it should be less severe, more spastic, and accompanied by hyperreflexia or myoclonus [31]. Fear of NMS should not prevent clinicians from prescribing antipsychotics in the street medicine setting, as its incidence is 0.01 to 0.02% of patients [29].

Catatonia Catatonia is a neuropsychiatric syndrome that is associated with antipsychotic medication, though it is unclear if the medication induces catatonia or reveals underlying predisposition to catatonia [32]. In fact, catatonia can occur after an antipsychotic is started, after an antipsychotic is withdrawn, and can occasionally be treated with an antipsychotic. Abnormal movements are a feature of catatonia, including rigidity, abnormal postures, repetitive purposeless movements, or lack of movement. Risk factors range from mood disorders and autism spectrum disorder to recent weight loss and cocaine use [33].

Catatonia can be stuporous, excited, or malignant. Malignant catatonia may include features of both stuporous and excited catatonia accompanied by autonomic instability and delirium. Psychotic explanations for not eating, such as poisoned food, should not fool you into removing catatonia from your differential diagnosis. Freely available online, the Bush-Francis Catatonia Rating Scale helps to rule in or out catatonia. Catatonia should be treated in the hospital with benzodiazepines and/or electroconvulsive therapy (ECT). If you suspect catatonia, you will likely need to involuntarily commit a patient with catatonia for inability to care for self, as they are typically unable to consent due to their symptoms and catatonia can lead to death if left untreated. The earlier treatment is initiated, the more successful it will be in reversing catatonia.

4.5.2.4 Sexual Dysfunction, Hyperprolactinemia, and Priapism

Antipsychotic-induced sexual dysfunction is common, regardless of gender, affecting between 30 and 80% of people taking them [34]. Sexual dysfunction includes decreased libido, erectile dysfunction, delayed orgasm, retrograde or painful ejaculation, amenorrhea, and disrupted menstrual cycles. Dopamine blockade causing hyperprolactinemia is implicated in the majority of cases, though antagonism of histamine, cholinergic, serotonin, and alpha-adrenergic receptors also play a role [35]. First generation antipsychotics, such as haloperidol (Haloperidol) and chlorpromazine (Thorazine), as well as risperidone and paliperidone more commonly cause sexual dysfunction than second generation prolactin-sparing antipsychotics such as aripiprazole (Abilify), quetiapine (Seroquel), clozapine (Clozaril), and ziprasidone (Geodon) [36]. Olanzapine (Zyprexa) can cause temporary hyperprolactinemia within the first six weeks of treatment, after which the prolactin level normalizes. Not uncommonly, men refuse risperidone and other antipsychotics because of news headlines of a lawsuit against Johnson and Johnson for risperidone-induced male breast enlargement and milk production [37]. However, hyperprolactinemia much more commonly causes other forms of sexual dysfunction listed at the beginning of this section.

Drawing labs to diagnose hyperprolactinemia can prove difficult in the street medicine setting. You may opt to skip the blood draw and move straight to treatment. Options include lowering the antipsychotic dose or switching to a prolactin-sparing antipsychotic. Alternatively, adding aripiprazole (Abilify) particularly if the patient cannot tolerate a lower dose or needs to be maintained on a prolactin-inducing antipsychotic for symptom control, can resolve hyperprolactinemia [38]. Start with 5 mg nightly. Aripiprazole has a high affinity for the dopamine receptor, knocking co-prescribed antipsychotics off the receptor. At higher doses of aripiprazole, psychosis symptoms may reemerge if aripiprazole is occupying too many of the dopamine receptors. While medications such as sildenafil (Viagra) improve antipsychotic-induced erectile dysfunction, it may be prohibitively expensive for street medicine patients and will not prevent long-term osteoporosis due to hyperprolactinemia.

Priapism Occurring in 0.5 to 0.9 per 100,000 cases annually in the United States, priapism is described as a painful erection lasting 4 h or more and is not associated with sexual arousal [39]. Overall, antipsychotics contribute little to the incidence of priapism, though they make up about 50% of the medication-induced ischemic priapism. Sickle cell anemia, prior priapism, and substance use disorders—predominantly cocaine, but also alcohol, methamphetamine, and narcotics—are associated with higher risk of priapism [40]. For individuals with these diagnoses, select among antipsychotics with lower alpha-1 affinity, as blockade of these receptors are implicated antipsychotic-induced priapism. Olanzapine (Zyprexa), aripiprazole (Abilify), haloperidol (Haldol) pose lower risk while chlorpromazine (Thorazine), ziprasidone (Geodon), and risperidone (Risperdal) are among the higher risk antipsychotics [41]. Counsel patients to go to the emergency room if priapism occurs; without treatment, permanent erectile dysfunction or impotence may occur.

4.5.2.5 Seizures

Antipsychotic medications cause seizures in approximately 0.04% of patients without epilepsy [42]. If a patient has a poorly controlled seizure disorder, consider starting an antiepileptic medication concurrently with the antipsychotic. Start with a low dose and monitor while slowly increasing the dose once weekly. Risperidone (Risperdal), quetiapine (Seroquel), and aripiprazole (Abilify) and first generation antipsychotics other than chlorpromazine (Thorazine), pose lower seizure risk for patients with epilepsy [43]. Select a lower risk antipsychotic for patients who currently drink alcohol and have a history of alcohol withdrawal seizures.

4.5.2.6 Overdose and Suicide

First- and second-generation antipsychotics have roughly the same risk of morbidity and mortality when taken in an overdose, though certain medications within each class vary with regard to mortality [44]. Overall mortality is low in overdose. Of second-generation antipsychotics, quetiapine (Seroquel), olanzapine (Zyprexa), and ziprasidone (Geodon) pose the highest risk for death in overdose due to respiratory depression with quetiapine and olanzapine and cardiac conduction problems with olanzapine and ziprasidone. Aripiprazole and lurasidone have the lowest studied morbidity and mortality at almost zero per 10,000 exposures [45]. Antipsychotics may lower the risk of suicidal ideation and suicidal attempts among people with schizophrenia and schizoaffective disorder. Clozapine is the only antipsychotic that specifically lowers suicide risk. Aripiprazole, olanzapine, and quetiapine have better evidence for lowering suicidal ideation and modest evidence for lowering suicidal behavior among patients with psychotic disorders. Some studies indicate that monotherapy with antipsychotics may increase the risk for suicide among patients with bipolar disorder, though the studies did not control for illness severity. When used as treatment for Major Depressive Disorder, quetiapine and aripiprazole may reduce suicidal ideation, though the evidence strength is lower for reducing suicide attempts [46].

4.6 Mood Stabilizers

Given the benefit for improvement of emotional lability and impulse control in the street medicine setting, the extended release valproic acid, divalproex ER (Depakote ER), and lamotrigine (Lamictal) are mood stabilizers worth considering for use in the street medicine setting within certain parameters. Lithium (multiple brand names), another mood stabilizer, should be avoided for someone sleeping outside. Most street mental health clinicians agree that prescribing lithium to someone sleeping rough is too risky due to its narrow therapeutic window, the need to draw labs, and the high likelihood of developing lithium toxicity with dehydration or concomitant nonsteroidal anti-inflammatory medications use. Carbamazepine (Tegretol) has the same benefits valproic acid, but it is more likely to cause agranulocytosis and dosing is complicated by the fact that it induces its own metabolism.

Divalproex ER (Depakote ER) is an antiepileptic with many years of research supporting its status as a gold-standard treatment for bipolar disorder. In the street medicine setting, clinicians have found it very helpful for improving mood lability and impulse control. Divalproex ER may also be helpful for treating mood lability and impulsivity among people diagnosed with both ADHD and epilepsy, though stimulants are first-line for ADHD [47]. Prescribing divalproex ER for patients who have cooccurring impulse control, mood lability, bipolar disorder, traumatic brain injury, seizures, migraines, or neuropathic pain may reduce pill burden, though valproic acid pills are enormous and cannot be cut or chewed. Lamotrigine is less useful in the setting of acute mania or depression with bipolar disorder because it takes nearly two months to reach a sufficient mood stabilizing dose. Lamotrigine is, however, the treatment of choice for behavioral symptoms of traumatic brain injury, good for migraine prophylaxis, and effective for absence seizures. Remember, if you are using divalproex ER or lamotrigine to treat bipolar disorder, it should control both mania and depression. If a patient continues to experience depression, increase the dose of the mood stabilizer if possible.

4.6.1 Mood Stabilizer Dosing

Because divalproex ER (Depakote ER) is lipophilic, the taller and wider the patient, the more medication they will need. The extended release form of valproic acid helps avoid significant gastrointestinal side effects and is dosed once daily. If your patient is prone to GI sensitivity or is very short and thin start, at 500 mg. Otherwise starting at 1000 mg is typically tolerated. The dose can be increased every 3–5 days up to 1500 mg depending on your patient's cognitive ability or your team's availability to provide observed doses. Aim for a divalproex ER dose of 1500 mg (or 1000 mg for short thin people) every evening prior for at least 5 days, then draw a level. Divalproex ER is typically given in the evening, as it is mildly sedating, but morning or mid-day dosing is also acceptable for many patients. If the trough level is below 50 mcg/mL, increase by 1000 mg and redraw the level in 1–2 weeks. Literature lists the therapeutic dose of valproic acid as 50–115 mcg/mL. Most patients tend to need an 80–100 mcg/mL level. In the street medicine setting, you may opt to dose based on symptom control rather than blood level while watching for mild symptoms of toxicity particularly in small people and at higher doses (over 2500–3000 mg daily). See Table 4.6 for additional dosing information.

Lamotrigine (Lamictal) should be dosed according to the package insert to avoid risk of Stevens Johnson syndrome. Aim for a total dose of 200–300 mg daily. Follow the dosing in Table U below carefully as a slow, lengthy titration reduces the risk. The lamotrigine package insert gives different dosing instructions for patients taking a variety of medications that interact with lamotrigine. Refer to it to avoid harm to your patient. If the patient stops taking lamotrigine for five or more days, they need to restart the titration. Often street mental health clinicians avoid prescribing lamotrigine because of its lengthy titration and risk of missed doses, though with the right patient and team resources, lamotrigine can be helpful and is a very well-tolerated mood stabilizer. Follow the same dosing instructions for behavioral symptoms of traumatic brain injury (TBI). Twice or three-times-daily dosing is preferred for TBI.

4.6.2 Laboratory Studies

Labs for lamotrigine are much simpler than valproic acid. For people who can become pregnant, complete a point-of-care urine pregnancy test prior to prescribing either medication to avoid neural tube defects in the fetus. Even if the patient is not sexually active, starting birth control before or at the same time as prescribing these mood stabilizers is worth considering given the risk of rape on the street. For valproic acid, ideally you can obtain aspartate transaminase (AST) and alanine transaminase (ALT) from a clinic or hospital within the past year prior to starting the medication. If unavailable, you can start valproic acid first, then check liver enzymes with the first valproic acid level check. Timing the blood draw at trough level is ideal, though you can estimate a trough level with a bit of math if you know when patient last took their medication. At 12–15 h after the last dose, the level will be 18 to 25% higher than it would be at trough [48]. Check the level only when the patient has been taking valproic acid for 5 days in a row unless you are concerned for toxicity. Ideally a complete blood count, transaminases, and valproic acid levels are checked at one month, three months, six months, and then yearly when the patient is on a stable dose. Depakote has a fairly wide therapeutic window, but can cause toxicity. In the street medicine setting, the likelihood of toxicity is low given inconsistent medication adherence. Observed dosing can also prevent toxicity if your team is able.

4.6.3 Mood Stabilizer Side Effects

Side effects of valproic acid include mild drowsiness, stomach upset, vomiting, diarrhea, hair loss or breakage, and tremor. Though headache is also listed as a side

Table 4.6 Mood stabilizer dosing

Name	Starting dose	Next dose	Next dose	Next dose	Next dose	Target dose
Valproic acid ER (Depakote ER)	500–1000 mg Qhs	1000–1500 mg Qhs	Check level or assess for mild toxicity before increasing	1500–2000 mg Qhs	2000–2500 mg Qhs	Aim for target trough level of 80–100 mcg/mL
Lamotrigine	25 mg Qam × 2 weeks	50 mg Qam × 2 weeks	100mg Qam × 2 weeks	150 mg Qam × 2 weeks	200 mg Qam	200–300 mg total per day

effect, valproic acid is a good option for migraine prophylaxis. Adverse effects include transaminase abnormalities and liver damage, fetal neural tube defects, thrombocytopenia, neutropenia, leukopenia, and pancytopenia. Other than neural tube defects, severe adverse effects are rare. Older age, gender assigned female at birth, and valproic acid levels above 80 mcg/mL in women are risk factors for thrombocytopenia, which occurs in five percent of people taking valproic acid [49].

Side effects of lamotrigine are typically mild and include rash, headache, mild sedation, insomnia, tremors, nausea, vomiting, and diarrhea. Most rashes associated with lamotrigine are benign and not a drug hypersensitivity reaction [49]. The major risk factors for the drug hypersensitivity rash are starting at a higher dose than 25 mg and increasing the dose too rapidly. Some people also have some genetic risk related to genetic polymorphisms encoding cytochrome P450 enzymes.

4.6.4 Valproic Acid Toxicity

Toxicity with divalproex ER occurs with intentional overdose or accidental overdose in the setting of liver impairment, high doses, supratherapeutic blood levels, rapid dose adjustments, or medication interactions. Mild toxicity occurs with overdoses of less than 200 mg/kg, moderate with doses of 200–400 mg/kg, and severe toxicity with greater than 800 mg/kg [50]. Mild symptoms can be managed by skipping 2–4 days of divalproex ER, then resuming at a lower dose. The higher the overdose, the more severe the symptoms and need for emergency intervention. Signs and symptoms of toxicity include fine tremors, ataxia, miosis, mild confusion, lethargy, tachycardia, vomiting, diarrhea, and abdominal pain. Patients with moderate to severe toxicity may develop hepatotoxicity or liver failure, hyperammonemic encephalopathy, arrhythmia, metabolic acidosis, hypernatremia, thrombocytopenia, and seizures. Severe toxicity may result in cerebral edema and herniation, multiorgan failure, coma, and death [51]. Despite the potential for toxicity with divalproex ER, it rarely occurs in street medicine practice. None of the authors of this handbook have seen a street medicine patient with toxicity in our collective 55 years of doing street medicine.

4.7 Antidepressants

If you determine that a patient has Major Depressive Disorder (MDD), PTSD, or any other anxiety disorder and your patient is interested in medication, prescribe an antidepressant. There are various antidepressant selection guides, treatment algorithms, personalized predictive algorithms using behavioral tests, and machine learning to assist in medication selection, titration, and switches. No major guides or algorithms account for the specific needs of people sleeping rough [52–55]. Some well-regarded tools, such as the Texas Medication Algorithm Project, use first-line medications that have questionable usefulness on the street, such as bupropion (Wellbutrin), buspirone (Buspar), and mirtazapine (Remeron) which are problematic for seizures and misuse, lengthy time to work, and sedation respectively. Even the landmark 2006 Sequenced Treatment Alternatives to Relieve Depression (STAR*D) trial has proven less impactful than initially hoped; a 2023 reanalysis of the STAR*D data shows remission rates were approximately half (35%) the originally published rate (67%) [56]. Other treatment algorithms include lifestyle changes and psychotherapy as major components of treatment, both of which are often inaccessible to street medicine patients.

4.7.1 Antidepressant Selection

Not all antidepressants have FDA approval for every anxiety disorder, but they all have the ability to treat MDD and anxiety disorders at the population level. At the individual level, however, there are multiple factors that make antidepressant medication selection difficult: individual genetics, other mental and physical health diagnoses, medication interactions, side effect profile, and tolerance. Erikson and colleagues suggest selecting a medication in collaboration with the patient, prioritizing safety, minimizing gastrointestinal and sedative side effects, and avoiding antidepressants with short half-lives that could cause antidepressant discontinuation syndrome for low-threshold treatment environments such as street medicine. They report that a serotonin reuptake inhibitor (SRI) or a serotonin norepinephrine reuptake inhibitor (SNRI) is a good first-line antidepressant option [57].

If a patient has taken an antidepressant in the past that worked well, discuss its safety profile for the street context and prescribe it if the patient prefers. An antidepressant that worked well for a close blood relative before may provide another good first-choice option. Close blood relatives share genetics and other characteristics with the patient that may offer insight into medications that are more effective. If the patient does not have information about family members' experiences with medications, antidepressant selection based on side effects offers the next best method of antidepressant selection. Time of day that the patient will remember to take the medication can also be an important factor. If they will typically remember to take it, but time may differ every day, select one of the medications listed as "alternatives" in the least sedating category below. Bupropion XL (Wellbutrin XL) should be prescribed for morning dosing and mirtazapine (Remeron) only at bedtime. Table 4.7 offers a quick reference for selection based on side effects and other considerations. See Sect. 4.7.7 below for full details of side effects. Medications are listed in alphabetical order, not by preference, level of effect, or any other quality. Keep in mind that individual patients may respond differently than the general population.

4.7.2 Antidepressant Dosing

Antidepressants are typically started at a low therapeutic level for Major Depressive Disorder and even lower for patients with anxiety disorders. This strategy works

Table 4.7 Initial medication selection quick reference (58–61)

Side effect/consideration	Medication options
Least sedating	First line: Bupropion XL (Wellbutrin XL), Fluoxetine (Prozac) Alternatives: Duloxetine (Cymbalta), Levomilnacipran (Fetzima), Sertraline (Zoloft) [58]
Fewest drug-drug interactions	Citalopram (Celexa), Desvenlafaxine (Pristiq), Escitalopram (Lexapro), Mirtazapine (Remeron), Venlafaxine XR (Effexor XR)
Least GI impact	First Line: Mirtazapine (Remeron) Alternatives: Bupropion XL (Wellbutrin XL), Citalopram (Celexa), Desvenlafaxine (Pristiq), Escitalopram (Lexapro), Fluoxetine (Prozac), Venlafaxine XR (Effexor XR)
Best cardiac profile	First line: Sertraline (Zoloft) Alternatives: Fluoxetine (Prozac), Paroxetine (Paxil)
Longest half-life, least likely to cause discontinuation syndrome	First line: Fluoxetine (Prozac) Alternatives: Bupropion XL (Wellbutrin XL), Citalopram (Celexa), Escitalopram (Lexapro), Levomilnacipran (Fetzima), Mirtazapine (Remeron), Vilazodone (Viibryd) Avoid: Paroxetine (Paxil), Venlafaxine XR (Effexor XR)
Least sexual side effects	First line: Bupropion XL (Wellbutrin XL), Desvenlafaxine (Pristiq), Mirtazapine (Remeron), Vilazodone (Viibryd), Vortioxetine (Trintellix) at lower doses Avoid: Paroxetine (Paxil)
Least weight gain	First line: Bupropion XL (Wellbutrin XL), Desvenlafaxine (Pristiq), Levomilnacipran (Fetzima), Vortioxetine (Trintellix) Alternatives: Fluoxetine (Prozac)
Lowers seizure threshold	Bupropion XL (Wellbutrin XL), tricyclic antidepressants
Pregnancy	First line: Sertraline (Zoloft) Alternatives: Citalopram (Celexa), Escitalopram (Lexapro), Fluoxetine (Prozac), Fluvoxamine (Luvox)
Best for chronic pain, neuropathic pain, migraines	Desvenlafaxine (Pristiq), Duloxetine (Cymbalta), Venlafaxine XR (Effexor XR) Avoid: Selective serotonin reuptake inhibitors (SSRI)

well for patients who are very anxious about side effects or who have experienced numerous side effects with antidepressants previously. Otherwise, a typical starting dose, whether the person is diagnosed with MDD, an anxiety disorder, or both, should be fine. Antidepressant doses can be increased as often as every two to four weeks. See Table 4.8 for additional dosing information for antidepressants.

Use the Patient Health Questionnaire-9 (PHQ-9), PTSD Checklist (PCL-5), Generalized Anxiety Disorder Questionnaire (GAD-7), or other questionnaire to measure symptoms and guide your decision to increase medication; regular use of patient-report questionnaires in behavioral health to guide treatment significantly improves treatment outcomes [62]. If the score has shown some improvement (two to four) points) in the first two weeks, wait a total of four weeks to change the medication dose. A clinically meaningful improvement in depression symptoms is five points or more on the PHQ-9 and GAD-7; aim for scores of less than 10. If you do not see this change in score, increase to the next dose as tolerated by the patient or consider switching the medication if necessary. If you are treating PTSD, a reduction in score by five to ten points shows promise and a reduction of 10-20 points is clinically meaningful [63]. Continue to increase the dose every two to four weeks until the patient has very few "quite a bit" and "extremely" scores on the PCL-5. When PTSD is in remission, all scores should be "a little bit" or "not at all."

Anxiety disorders tend to require higher doses of antidepressants than depressive disorders for response and remission. While remission of depression and anxiety disorders may not be possible in the street medicine context, street psychiatrists routinely observe clinically meaningful symptom reduction with treatment despite the patient's circumstances. Avoid the trap that some clinicians fall into of blaming the symptoms on the patient's living environment and therefore not increasing medication doses or switching medications when indicated. Some providers are uncomfortable with prescribing high doses of antidepressants. If you are one of these clinicians, work to improve your comfort level in order to be an effective prescriber for your patient.

Within the street medicine context, you may find that patients respond better to antidepressant treatment than you expect from medication alone. The impact of loneliness and stigma on the mental well-being of people living unsheltered is unsurprisingly massive. The love and respect street medicine teams can offer provides patients with emotional support that measurably improves their mental well-being [64]. Medication and unconditional love can be a powerful combination.

4.7.3 Switching Antidepressants

Consider a change of medications if the patient has not achieved significant improvement in symptoms at the highest dose or cannot tolerate the side effects at an effective dose. Early improvement within the first two to four weeks, has good positive predictive value for achieving remission or greatly improved symptoms. However, as many as 25% of patients who do not have any improvement by week four will still go on to achieve good outcomes [65]. Patients who have not reached remission or a great improvement of symptoms after 16 weeks of taking the same antidepressant should be encouraged to switch antidepressants. An antidepressant within the same class, such as changing from one SSRI to another, may work well if side effects are the reason for switching. If ineffectiveness necessitates a medication switch, try a different class of antidepressants, such as switching from a SSRI to a SNRI.

Typically, clinicians cross-titrate antidepressants in making the switch, as it is better tolerated by most patients. The chaos of the streets and cognitive impairment of people living there presents a challenge to cross-titration in the street medicine environment. Rely on your knowledge of the patient, the patient's preference, and the likelihood of discontinuation syndrome in the decision to stop an antidepressant cold turkey to switch or to cross-titrate. Patients with impaired cognition may fare better with the cold turkey switch as might patients who have never had discontinuation syndrome from previous antidepressant trials. Patients with good cognition or those who have experienced discontinuation syndrome even with antidepressants with longer half-lives will do better with a cross-titration.

Your team's ability to see the patient more frequently, such as every few days to a week, can improve your patient's ability to successfully cross-titrate as well. Some prescribers prefer a cross-titration over the course of two to three months to minimize discontinuation syndrome, but in the context of the streets three months is a lifetime. Cross-titrations over the course of a month for cognitively organized patients is often the longest cross-titration feasible on the streets. Many psychiatric providers do not prescribe paroxetine (Paxil) or venlafaxine XR (Effexor XR) on the streets due to the severity of discontinuation syndrome with these antidepressants and the several months or more required to cross-titrate.

4.7.4 Antidepressant Augmentation

If an antidepressant is partially effective, but insufficient to produce significant treatment response or remission, augmentation with another medication may be helpful. Because less is more with street pharmacology, you may opt to use augmentation less often. Medications such as buspirone, bupropion, mirtazapine, and trazodone can be safely and effectively combined with other antidepressants, though you will need to weigh their risks and benefits in the street medicine setting [66]. Avoid combinations of two SSRIs or two SNRIs as well as combinations of a SSRI or SNRI with tricyclic antidepressants and monoamine oxidase inhibitors due to the potential of side effects and serotonin syndrome. Tricyclic antidepressants, such as amitriptyline (Elavil), and monoamine oxidase inhibitors, such as selegiline (Emsam), are typically too risky to prescribe to people sleeping outside because of side effects, problems in combination with certain foods, and toxicity in overdose. For anxious patients or patients with PTSD, augmentation with hydroxyzine (Atarax), propranolol, and prazosin may be helpful. See Table 4.9 for dosing information for augmentation medications not listed in Table 4.8. Some psychiatrists combine antidepressants and low-dose antipsychotics for augmentation of depression.

There is a caveat for antidepressant augmentation: adding a medication specifically for sleep or anxiety at any time during the course of antidepressant treatment may be warranted. For example, some clinicians add hydroxyzine (Atarax) during the first two to four weeks when starting an antidepressant if the patient needs a faster-acting medication for anxiety. Hydroxyzine can cause mild sedation, though less than medications such as mirtazapine and trazodone. Because antidepressants can take a few weeks to start working, this strategy may be helpful for patients who want something to help them feel better now. Hydroxyzine can cause mild sedation, though less than medications like mirtazapine (Remeron) and trazodone (Desyrel).

Trazodone is a helpful medication for sleep, as is diphenhydramine (Benadryl), as long as the patient wants to take a sedative medication. Diphenhydramine (Benadryl) and hydroxyzine (Atarax) are both anticholinergic and can be problematic with older individuals with cognitive dysfunction. Propranolol (Inderal) can be taken at doses of 10 to 20 mg as needed for social or performance anxiety or daily at the same low doses for generalized anxiety. Clonidine (Catapres) is used in

Table 4.8 Antidepressant medication dosing [58]

Medication	Starting dose	Next dose	Next dose	Next dose	Max dose	Other
Amitriptyline	50 mg Qhs	75 mg Qhs	100 mg Qhs	125 mg Qhs	150 mg Qhs	
Bupropion XL (Wellbutrin XL)	150 mg Qam	300 mg Qam	450 mg Qam	None	450 mg Qam	Avoid SR formulation
Citalopram (Celexa)	20 mg Qhs	30 mg Qhs	40 mg Qhs	None	40 mg Qhs	Extra QTc risk above 40 mg
Desvenlafaxine (Pristiq)	50 mg Qam or Qhs	100 mg Qam or Qhs	None	None	100 mg Qam or Qhs	Most people only need 50 mg daily
Duloxetine (Cymbalta)	30 mg Qam or Qhs	60 mg Qam or Qhs	90 mg Qam or Qhs	120 mg Qam or Qhs	120 mg Qam or Qhs	
Escitalopram (Lexapro)	10 mg Qhs	20 mg Qhs	30 mg Qhs	40 mg Qhs	40 mg Qhs	Rarely needed >30 mg Qhs
Fluoxetine (Prozac)	20 mg Qam	40 mg Qam	60 mg Qam	80 mg Qam	80 mg Qam	Rarely needed >60 mg Qam
Fluvoxamine (Luvox)	50 mg Qhs	100 mg Qhs	150 mg Qhs	50 mg Qam + 150 mg Qhs	150 mg BID	Divide doses above 150 mg
Levominalcipran (Fetzima)	20 mg Qam	40 mg Qam	80 mg Qam	120 mg Qam	120 mg Qam	Give 20 mg for 2 days, then 40 mg daily
Mirtazapine (Remeron)	15 mg Qhs	30 mg Qhs	45 mg Qhs	None	45 mg Qhs	
Paroxetine (Paxil)	20 mg Qhs	40 mg Qhs	50 mg Qhs	60 mg Qhs	60 mg Qhs	Max dose may need prior authorization
Sertraline (Zoloft)	50 mg Qam or Qhs	100 mg Qam or Qhs	150 mg Qam or Qhs	200 mg Qam or Qhs	200 mg Qam or Qhs	
Venlafaxine XR (Effexor XR)	37.5 mg Qhs	75 mg Qhs	150 mg Qhs	225 mg Qhs	300 mg Qhs	Divided doses may work better for pain
Vilazodone (Viibryd)	10 mg Qam or Qhs	20 mg Qam or Qhs	40 mg Qam or Qhs	none	40 mg Qam or Qhs	Increase to 20 mg after 1 week
Vortioxetine (Trintellix)	5 mg Qam or Qhs	10 mg Qam or Qhs	15 mg Qam or Qhs	20 mg Qam or Qhs	20 mg Qam or Qhs	

psychiatry for anxiety, though given its risk of hypotension and rebound hypertension, the transdermal patch is safer for the streets than pills. Use caution when prescribing clonidine in communities where it is used as part of a street drug cocktail.

Prazosin can be helpful for patients with nightmares related to PTSD. If patients with PTSD complain of poor sleep, prazosin may help regardless if the person remembers having nightmares or not. Some patients report waking up sweaty with a racing pulse, but do not remember a nightmare. Prazosin (Minipress) can be given

Table 4.9 Augmentation dosing

Medication	Starting dose	Next dose	Next dose	Next dose	Max dose	Other
Clonidine (Catapres) transdermal patch	0.1 mg Q7 days	0.2 mg Q7 days	0.3 mg Q7 days	none	0.3 mg Q7 days	Closely monitor blood pressure. Clean skin prior to affixing patch.
Buspirone (Buspar)	5–10 mg Qhs	10 mg BID	20 mg BID	20 mg TID	30 mg TID	Takes a long time to work. Do not use PRN
Hydroxyzine (Atarax)	10–25 mg once daily scheduled or PRN	10–25 mg BID scheduled or PRN	10–25 mg TID scheduled or PRN	50 mg BID—TID scheduled or PRN	50 mg QID scheduled or PRN	Vistaril and Atarax are both brand names for hydroxyzine. Atarax comes in a tablet and can be given at smaller doses than Vistaril
Prazosin	1 mg Qhs	2 mg Qhs	3 mg Qhs	4 mg Qhs	16+ mg Qhs	Dose may be increased every 2–3 nights until nightmares reduce or cease
Propranolol	10 mg once daily scheduled or PRN	20 mg once daily scheduled or PRN	20 mg twice daily scheduled or PRN	none	20 mg twice daily scheduled or PRN	Most patients do not need more than 20 mg daily
Trazodone (Desyrel)	25–50 mg Qhs	100 mg Qhs	150 mg Qhs	200 mg Qhs	300 mg Qhs	Max dose recommended for sleep/ augmentation on the street

Qam every morning; Qhs every evening; Q7 every seven; BID twice/day; TID three times/day; QID four times/day

at a wide range of doses, though it will cause lower blood pressure and dizziness for some people at higher doses. Most providers use a maximum dose of 16 mg nightly, though doses as high as 30 to 45 mg nightly have been used safely and effectively among adults with severe PTSD-related nightmares. Check with the patient's primary care provider before starting propranolol (Inderal), clonidine (Catapres), or prazosin (Minipress) if they are taking other antihypertensives.

There are few anxiolytics as effective as benzodiazepines. However, they are not recommended for PTSD and due their lethality when combined with opioids, prescribing them is risky in the street medicine setting. Benzodiazepines are not recommended for PTSD because they improve a person's ability to avoid all thoughts and feelings related to trauma. Avoidance itself is a symptom of PTSD and PTSD will worsen with further avoidance. If you decide to prescribe a benzodiazepine on the streets, mitigate risk by giving a low dose and time-limited (one week or less) prescription. Other medications used to treat anxiety disorders include antidepressants, propranolol, clonidine, gabapentin, prazosin, hydroxyzine pamoate, and buspirone. In some places, gabapentin and clonidine have a street value and some people develop gabapentin use disorder. Oral clonidine can cause risky extremes of blood pressure and is safer as a patch when used to treat anxiety. Otherwise, non-benzodiazepine anxiolytics have a good safety profile on the streets.

4.7.5 Stopping an Antidepressant

Guidelines vary in their recommendations for how long after remission of a depressive episode to wait until discontinuing the antidepressant, suggesting 4 to 12 months if at all [67]. Return of subsequent episodes of depression is high; the lifetime risk of a recurrent episode is 60% after one episode, 70% after two episodes, and 90% after three episodes [68]. Cooccurring disorders, such as PTSD, may also warrant continued treatment with antidepressants. Most street medicine patients will not reach sufficient remission of symptoms while sleeping outside to warrant stopping the antidepressant and many will have had multiple past depressive episodes. However, if your patient needs to stop taking antidepressants or wants to stop, knowing how to minimize risk with discontinuation is helpful.

The two major risks with antidepressant discontinuation are return of depressive symptoms and discontinuation syndrome. Patients are at highest risk of relapse during the first two months after discontinuing an antidepressant [69]. Tapering antidepressants slowly over two weeks or longer reduces the risk of relapse for depression and several anxiety disorders [70]. The next section on antidepressant discontinuation syndrome (ADS) provides information on preventing and treating ADS symptoms.

4.7.6 Antidepressant Discontinuation Syndrome (ADS)

Street medicine clinicians rarely see ADS among people sleeping outside compared to the estimated incidence of ADS of 15–56% in research [71]. Risk factors for ADS include short half-life of the antidepressant, gender assigned female at birth, younger age, experiencing adverse effects early in treatment, higher doses or longer duration of medication treatment, abrupt cessation of an antidepressant, history of discontinuation syndrome, genetic variations in the serotonin 1A receptor [72, 73]. Theories about the discrepancy in incidence observed in street medicine patients include reduced risk due to adherence difficulties, avoidance of antidepressants with short half-lives by street medicine providers, and attributing ADS symptoms to other causes, and general poor health causing people sleeping rough not to notice milder symptoms. One former street medicine patient described her experience of ADS from venlafaxine XR (Effexor XR) as similar to withdrawal from heroin or fentanyl.

Nevertheless, the discontinuation syndrome has the ability to occur with nearly every antidepressant, possibly with the exception of fluoxetine (Prozac). Symptoms of ADS include flu-like symptoms of nausea, headache, fatigue, arthralgias and myalgias. Electric shock or zap sensations are also commonly described. Patients may also have restlessness, agitation, insomnia, irritability, anxiety, confusion, palpitations, dizziness, and sweating. A 2019 study suggests that current US and UK guidelines for antidepressant discontinuation syndrome grossly underestimate the severity and length of discontinuation symptoms [74].

There are several methods for preventing and treating ADS. Avoid prescribing Paroxetine (Paxil) and venlafaxine XR (Effexor XR) in the street setting unless absolutely necessary for the patient's mental well-being. When planning to discontinue an antidepressant, make sure your patient is still actually taking it. If so, you may opt to slowly taper their antidepressant over weeks to possibly months or switch to fluoxetine (Prozac), as its active metabolite auto-tapers with a half-life of 7 to 15 days. Case studies suggest to start fluoxetine 20 to 40 mg daily and stop the patient's other antidepressant, continue fluoxetine for 7 days, then discontinue fluoxetine [75]. Use caution with this method, as fluoxetine interacts with many other medications. Treat milder symptoms with over-the-counter medications. If moderate to severe symptoms occur during a slow taper, increase to the dose that did not cause symptoms and taper more slowly. If you have to taper someone off paroxetine (Paxil), the liquid formulation offers smaller dose adjustments. Venlafaxine XR (Effexor XR) can be switched to regular-release venlafaxine at low doses to provide an easier discontinuation.

4.7.7 Antidepressant Side Effects, Adverse Effects, and Their Management

Most antidepressants are well tolerated. Unfortunately, most side effects occur within the first two weeks and positive effects of antidepressants often take more than two weeks to appear. The best management strategy is letting the patient know what to expect before prescribing the medication, then providing encouragement or support to continue taking the medication while waiting for the side effects to resolve. Equally, giving patients permission in advance to stop a medication they cannot tolerate will relieve anxiety for most patients surrounding side effects. This permission also helps your patient feel comfortable telling you they are not taking or intermittently taking their antidepressant without fear of judgment. Address concerns about sexual side effects and weight gain prior to starting the medication, as most people will have heard about these side effects and they do not improve over time. Because there are so many different antidepressant options, reassure your patient you will likely be able to find an alternative if one of these side effects occur.

Side effect comparisons between antidepressants are listed in Table 4.10. Given the relative safety of other antidepressant options, tricyclic antidepressants and monoamine oxidase inhibitors are not recommended for street medicine. Amitriptyline (Elavil), a tricyclic antidepressant, is included in Table 4.10 to demonstrate the safety risks with tricyclics and is not recommended for street-based treatment. The overdose risks listed in Table 4.10 are out of a total of 10,000 deaths. While the actual number of overdose deaths is low, even for amitriptyline, a

Table 4.10 Antidepressant side effect comparison [45, 58, 76–79]

Medication	GI	Sedation	Weight gain	Sexual effects	Overdose risk	Cardiac risk	Seizure risk
Amitriptyline	++	+++	++	++	++++	++++	++
Bupropion XL (Wellbutrin XL)	+	– –	– –	–	++	+ HTN/P	C
Citalopram (Celexa)	+	+	++	++	++	+QTc	+
Desvenlafaxine (Pristiq)	+	+	–	+	++	+HTN	–
Duloxetine (Cymbalta)	++	–	++	–	+	+OH	–
Escitalopram (Lexapro)	+	+	++	++	–	+QTc	+
Fluoxetine (Prozac)	+	– –	+	++	–	–	–
Fluvoxamine (Luvox)	++	+	+	++	++	–	–?
Levominalcipran (Fetzima)	++	–	–	+++	–	++++	+?
Mirtazapine (Remeron)	–	+++[a]	+++[a]	++?	+	–	+
Paroxetine (Paxil)	++	++	++	+++	–	–	+
Sertraline (Zoloft)	++	+	+	++	–	–	+
Venlafaxine XR (Effexor XR)	+	+/–	+	++	++	++ HTN/P	+
Vilazodone (Viibryd)	+++	–	+	+/–	–	–?	++?
Vortioxetine (Trintellix)	++	+	–	See below[b]	–	–?	–

– – opposite effect; – minimal/no effect; + mild effect; ++ moderate effect; +++ marked effect ++++ extremely risky, avoid use; ? insufficient evidence; *C* contraindicated; *HTN* hypertension; *P* pulse; *OH* orthostatic hypotension

[a]Worse at lower doses

[b]Vilazodone sexual side effects are dose dependent with minimal effect at low doses and at effects similar to most SSRIs at higher doses

15-30 day supply can result in death. Four plus signs (++++) indicates over 20 deaths; three (+++) indicates 10–19 deaths; ++ indicates 4–9 deaths; + indicates 2–4 deaths, and—indicates less than two deaths per 10,000.

Note that Table 4.10 is the author's best estimate of comparisons as there is some controversy, conflicting, and missing information in studies of antidepressants. Risk comparisons should not be drawn between antipsychotics and antidepressants based on the tables in this chapter. Each table only demonstrates within-class comparisons, despite the use of the same symbols.

4.7.7.1 Sedation

Most antidepressants cause mild sedation at most with the exception of mirtazapine (Remeron) and trazodone (Desyrel). Mirtazapine is most sedating at doses of 7.5 to 15 mg and less sedating at higher doses. In comparison to antipsychotics, antidepressants as a class are far less sedating. Many antidepressants can be taken at any time of day, though paroxetine, venlafaxine, citalopram, and escitalopram tend to be prescribed at bedtime.

4.7.7.2 Gastrointestinal (GI) Effects

Waiting is the general recommendation for GI side effects of antidepressants, as they usually dissipate within the first two weeks. If stomach upset occurs, taking the antidepressant with food and staying hydrated will reduce symptoms. Start at a lower dose and consider a time-limited supply of supportive medications for patients who do not want to try an antidepressant due to past GI side effects. Over-the-counter medications such as loperamide (Imodium), bismuth subsalicylate (Pepto-Bismol), calcium carbonate (Tums), and simethicone (Gas-X) typically suffice for GI discomfort with antidepressants. Odansetron (Zofran), a prescription medication, may be helpful for patients prone to nausea.

4.7.7.3 Weight Gain

If weight gain is a concern for your patient or has been problematic in the past, avoid mirtazapine (Remeron). Citalopram (Celexa), Duloxetine (Cymbalta), Escitalopram (Lexapro), and paroxetine (Paxil) also tend to cause more weight gain than other antidepressants. Rough sleeping populations may walk more than the general population and may be at less risk of weight gain with antidepressants. However, because lifestyle changes are often inaccessible for street medicine patients, the best option to mitigate weight gain is to prescribe less offending antidepressants.

4.7.7.4 Sexual Dysfunction

Sexual dysfunction is common among people with depression, with over 40% of untreated men and 50% of untreated women experiencing reduced sexual interest. Street medicine patients also often have comorbid physical health problems that cause sexual dysfunction. Make sure to assess sexual dysfunction prior to initiating an antidepressant, as patients may blame the antidepressant rather than preexisting conditions. Equally, once the patient starts an antidepressant, ask them about sexual side effects, as they often result in nonadherence and patients tend not to report sexual side effects on their own.

A comprehensive literature review in 2017 found that SSRIs cause sexual dysfunction more than other antidepressants because of their serotonergic effects [80]. The most common SSRI sexual side effects are delayed ejaculation and female orgasm, though reduced libido, erectile dysfunction, anorgasmia, and reduced sexual satisfaction also occur [81]. Sexual side effects tend to be dose-dependent and reversible with very few patients reporting them after SSRI discontinuation. Bupropion, mirtazapine, or SNRIs work best for patients concerned about sexual dysfunction [35]. Venlafaxine XR (Effexor XR), however, has sexual side effects similar to SSRIs, possibly because it has more serotonergic properties than other SNRIs. For patients who need SSRIs, bupropion XL may be added to counteract sexual dysfunction, though its risks among people sleeping outside should be considered. Other options to reduce the sexual impact of antidepressant include lowering the dose, as the effects are usually dose-dependent.

Phosphodiesterase-5 inhibitors, such as sildenafil (Viagra) and tadalafil (Cialis), may be appropriate for some patients assigned male and female at birth, though cost may prevent their use in the street medicine setting [82, 83]. Phosphodiesterase-5 inhibitors are not FDA-approved for sexual dysfunction in people assigned female at birth.

4.7.7.5 Suicidal Ideation

The Food and Drug Administration (FDA) added a black box warning to all antidepressants warning that antidepressant medications can increase suicidal thoughts and behaviors in some individuals ages 25 and younger. The FDA subsequently added that depression can also cause these symptoms. The American Psychiatric Association, in 2025, noted the harms of untreated depression for people within this age group, reporting that completed suicides increased after the FDA warning was added [84]. Fornaro and colleagues suggest frequent follow-up and the inclusion of other caregivers in the initial phase of antidepressant treatment [85]. Street medicine teams can reduce risk for patients ages 25 and younger by evaluating suicidal ideation prior to prescribing, prescribing antidepressants with low risk with overdose, enlisting the support of friends or family on the street, and checking in with the patient more often within the first one to two months of initiating an antidepressant. Phone call check-ins about suicidal ideation are acceptable. If your team is only able to see the patient once monthly, the risk of untreated depression is likely higher than the risk of prescribing a low starting dose of an antidepressant with follow-up in one month.

4.7.7.6 Headaches and Migraines

Headache, similar to sexual dysfunction, is a more common SSRI side effect than other antidepressants. Non-migraine headaches are most prominent within the first two weeks of treatment and tend to improve with time. Acetaminophen may be safer with SSRI-related headaches in patients prone to bleeding, as SSRIs and nonsteroidal anti-inflammatory medications both increase risk of bleeding. Migraines, however, have a bidirectional relationship with depression: depression itself can cause migraines and migraines can cause depression [86]. Similarly, some anxiety disorders are also associated with headaches, obsessive compulsive disorder in particular [87]. Medications that treat both migraines and depression include desvenlafaxine (Pristiq), duloxetine (Cymbalta), venlafaxine XR (Effexor XR), and tricyclic antidepressants. Of these, desvenlafaxine and duloxetine may be preferred in the street medicine setting.

4.7.7.7 Seizures

The only medication contraindicated in patients with a history of seizures is bupropion, though tricyclic antidepressants pose substantial risk as well. Different studies show some with other antidepressants, though the overall risk of antidepressants is quite low, even among people with epilepsy [88]. This 2017 systematic review recommends fluoxetine (Prozac) and duloxetine (Cymbalta) as having almost no risk for patients with epilepsy and concluded that citalopram (Celexa), escitalopram (Lexapro), mirtazapine (Remeron), paroxetine (Paxil), and sertraline (Zoloft) have a low to moderate risk. A 2015 study found that over five years, 0.37% of general primary care patients had new-onset seizures [89]. This study suggests avoiding venlafaxine and trazodone for patients with substantial risk of seizures. There are very few studies comparing antidepressants that include vilazodone (Viibryd) and levomilnacipran (Fetzima). The FDA label for prescribing levomilnacipran notes that seizures can occur. There are case reports of breakthrough seizures among patients taking vilazodone (Viibryd) with previously controlled epilepsy [90].

4.7.7.8 Serotonin Syndrome

Serotonin syndrome is an uncommon adverse effect of antidepressants and other serotonergic agents, which ranges from mild to life-threatening. Symptoms typically start within 24 h of introducing a new serotonergic medication or substance, increasing the dose, or changes that alter the metabolism of a serotonergic agent. In addition to antidepressants and some antipsychotics, substances such as cocaine, ecstasy (MDMA), dextromethorphan, opiates, and LSD have serotonergic effects. Symptoms of serotonin syndrome include sweating, flushing, goosebumps, vomiting, diarrhea, increased bowel sounds, dilated pupils, hyperreflexia, autonomic instability (most commonly tachycardia and hypertension), muscle rigidity, myoclonus, agitation, restlessness, confusion, and insomnia. Life-threatening signs include high fever, seizure, arrhythmias, and unconsciousness. Though incidence is difficult to quantify, only 0.18% of toxic exposures to SSRIs resulted in death [31]. The differential diagnosis includes neuroleptic malignant syndrome, anticholinergic toxicity, malignant hyperthermia, and sympathomimetic toxicity. It may be impossible to distinguish between serotonin syndrome and sympathomimetic toxicity, as many sympathomimetics increase serotonin levels. Table 4.11 below distinguishes some of the differences in toxidromes.

Table 4.11 Differences in toxidromes similar to serotonin syndrome

Toxidrome	Cause	Onset	Predominant neuromuscular findings	Bowel sounds
Serotonin syndrome	Serotonergic agents (antidepressants, 2nd generation antipsychotics, others)	Within 24 h of starting, adding, increasing the dose of a serotonergic agent	Neuromuscular hyperactivity (hyperreflexia, tremor, spasticity, myoclonus, clonus)	Hyperactive
Neuroleptic malignant syndrome	Dopamine antagonists (antipsychotics) or dopamine withdrawal	Days to weeks; idiosyncratic and not dose- dependent	Neuromuscular hypoactivity (cogwheeling, bradykinesia, lead-pipe rigidity)	Hypoactive
Anticholinergic toxicity	Anticholinergic agents	Sudden, less than 24 h	Sometimes normal muscle tone and reflexes; may have clonus	Hypoactive
Sympatho-mimetic Toxicity	Stimulants (amphetamine, methamphetamine, cocaine, MDMA, bath salts)	Within 24 h of ingestion	Increased muscle tone, hyperreflexia	Hypoactive or absent

4.8 Treatment for ADHD

The treatment of choice for ADHD in adults is stimulants [91]. In the guidelines for treating stimulant use disorders, the American Society of Addiction Medicine (ASAM) and the American Academy of Addiction Psychiatry (AAAP) recommend considering treating ADHD with stimulants even in the setting of a stimulant use disorder [92]. Non-stimulants options exist, but are typically less efficacious compared to stimulants. This appears to be particularly true in the street medicine setting where patients often have tried to treat their ADHD with methamphetamine (meth) or cocaine.

4.8.1 Stimulant Medications for ADHD

Though there are risks with stimulant medications for ADHD, they are generally lower than the risk of remaining homeless because of untreated or poorly treated ADHD. Prescribed stimulants are typically "a drop in the bucket" compared to the health risks of using meth or cocaine/crack. Each patient is different and you should use your best clinical judgment, particularly in patients with decompensated congestive heart failure (CHF) and untreated psychosis. Psychiatric providers typically treat psychosis first before starting a stimulant. If the patient stops using meth and the psychosis abates, you may try lowering the dose slowly. Without meth, the patient may do well on a lower antipsychotic dose or may not need an antipsychotic. Careful monitoring of benefits versus harms is important throughout treatment. Though research is mixed on the usefulness of prescribed stimulants to treat methamphetamine use disorder, some street clinicians have noted that their patients treated with prescribed stimulants for ADHD are frequently able to reduce their use of meth and cocaine. You may consider this possibility in weighing the risks and benefits of stimulants; if a prescribed stimulant can help lower the use of street stimulants, prescribing a stimulant may actually be the less harmful option in the setting of psychosis and CHF.

If you have the ability, ASAM recommends trying a longer acting stimulant first, such as extended release methylphenidate products (Ritalin LA, Concerta, Focalin XR) or extended release amphetamine products (Adderall XR, Vyvanse). In the United States, stimulants used to treat adults with ADHD often require a prior authorization if the person has insurance. Some public insurance plans require urine drug screen (UDS) results prior to authorizing a stimulant and often they will not authorize longer acting stimulants without a trial of shorter acting stimulants first. Methylphenidate and mixed amphetamine salts are typically preferred by Medicaid, as these shorter acting products. In my practice, patients tend to prefer the shorter acting stimulants and have no difficulty dosing them multiple times per day. Once they have taken the shorter-acting stimulant first, it can be difficult to switch to a longer-acting stimulant without breaking trust. Further, evidence suggests that immediate release stimulants are superior to long-acting stimulants in symptom control. One meta-analysis demonstrated that the clinical benefit of immediate-release methylphenidate (Ritalin) among adults is 3.26 times greater than longer-acting stimulants and was the only medication demonstrating improvement of ADHD symptoms in patients with cooccurring substance use disorders [93].

In the U.S., almost all stimulants require prior authorizations from Medicaid and some Medicaid providers require urine drug screen results prior to authorizing stimulants. Rules requiring urine drug screens are largely applied in the United States to poor populations with public insurance and not to patients who can afford private insurance. These rules are antiquated and are not consistent with medical guidelines for treating ADHD in the setting of a stimulant use disorder. If a UDS is required for authorization, have your patient provide a urine sample at a time they know no methamphetamine will be in their urine. Some street psychiatrists will throw away a UDS positive for meth or cocaine without recording it in the medical record when attempting to obtain a negative screen for insurance purposes. Patients may need to try multiple times to obtain a negative UDS. Positives for other substances do not appear to result in a denial of authorization for prescription stimulants.

4.8.1.1 Stimulant Selection

When selecting a stimulant to try, one that worked before is likely to work again. If the patient has not tried a stimulant before, there is no clear better choice between methylphenidate products and amphetamine products. Some studies and guidelines recommend methylphenidate first citing better efficacy, while other studies recommend amphetamine products first due to better tolerability [94, 95]. Practically, if you plan to confirm your patient is taking the stimulant you prescribed, most urine drug screens test for amphetamines but not all screen for methylphenidate. You may have to order different cups or cups with a larger panel of substances to be able to test for methylphenidate products or have access to a lab that will test for it. If your team only has enough money to buy UDS cups without methylphenidate, there is no harm in only prescribing amphetamine products until you have the capacity to comfortably prescribe methylphenidate.

4.8.1.2 Stimulant Dosing

Expect to need to increase the dose, potentially to the highest dose for your street medicine patients to have improvement of ADHD symptoms. You can increase the dose at weekly intervals as needed to improve symptoms. Try the maximum tolerable dose (the dose at which side effects are absent or manageable) before determining the stimulant will not work. Even if the stimulant is not working at all at lower doses, it may work at higher doses. The ASAM/AAAP stimulant use disorder guidelines indicate that the maximum dose is often needed to adequately treat cocaine and methamphetamine use disorders. For street medicine patients with cooccurring vADHD and stimulant use disorder, you may need to follow the ASAM/AAAP guidance on dosing for best efficacy. Use your clinical judgment when managing benefits compared to negative effects in patients with challenging comorbid conditions such as CHF or psychosis.

See Table 4.12 below for short, intermediate, and longer acting methylphenidate products used to treat ADHD and their dosing. See Table 4.13 below for

Table 4.12 Methylphenidate medications for ADHD [96, 97]

Medication and available strengths	Duration of action	Starting dose	Next dose	Next dose	Max dose
Methylphenidate (Ritalin)	3–4 h	5 mg BID	10 mg BID	20 mg BID	30 mg BID
Methylphenidate HCl (Methylin)	3–4 h	5 mg BID	10 mg BID	20 mg BID	30 mg BID
Dexmethylphenidate (Focalin)	3–4 h	2.5 mg BID	5 mg BID	5 mg Qam, 2.5 mg every afternoon	10 mg BID
Sustained release methylphenidate (Ritalin SR)	4–8 h	20 mg Qam	40 mg Qam	60 mg Qam	60 mg Qam
Methylphenidate HCl extended release (Methylin ER, Metadate ER, Ritalin LA)[a]	4–12 h	20 mg Qam	30–40 mg Qam	50–60 mg Qam	60 mg Qam
Methylphenidate HCl extended release (Concerta)	12 h	18 mg Qam	27 mg Qam	36 mg Qam	54 mg Qam

[a]Various brand name methylphenidate HCl extended release brand names contain varying mixtures of short and long-acting methylphenidate, causing their duration of action to vary

Table 4.13 Amphetamine products for ADHD [96–98]

Medication and available strengths	Duration of action	Starting dose	Next dose	Next dose	Max dose
Dextroamphetamine (Dexedrine) 5 mg	3–5 h	5 mg BID	10 mg BID	15 mg BID	20 mg BID
Dextroamphetamine (Dextrostat) 5, 10 mg	3–5 h	5 mg BID	10 mg BID	15 mg BID	20 mg BID
Methamphetamine (Desoxyn) 5 mg	3–5 h	5 mg BID	10 mg BID	None	10 mg BID
Mixed amphetamine salts or dextroamphetamine + amphetamine (Adderall) 5, 10, 20, 30 mg	4–8 h	5–10 mg BID	20 mg BID	20 mg TID or 30 mg BID	60 mg total daily
Dextroamphetamine sulfate (Dexedrine spansules) 5, 10, 15 mg	8–12 h	10 mg Qam or 5 mg BID	15–20 mg Qam or 10 mg BID	20–30 mg Qam or 10–15 mg BID	60 mg Qam or divided BID or TID
Extended release mixed amphetamine salts (Adderall XR) 5, 10, 15, 20, 25, 30 mg	8–12 h	5–10 mg Qam	15–20 mg Qam	20–25 mg Qam	30 mg Qam
Extended release mixed amphetamine salts (Mydayis ER)	8–12 h	12.5 mg Qam	25 mg Qam	37.5 mg Qam	50 mg Qam
Lisdexamphetamine (Vyvanse) 10, 20, 30, 40, 50, 60, 70 mg	14 h	30 mg Qam	40–50 mg Qam	50–70 mg qam	70 mg Qam

amphetamine products and their dosing. Chewable tablets, transdermal patches, and liquid formulations of several medications exist, if needed for patients, that are not included in the tables. Twice daily (BID) dosing in this chart means morning and early afternoon dosing, not morning and evening.

Longer-acting stimulants may not sufficiently control symptoms during the day. Pediatricians and psychiatric providers commonly prescribe an early afternoon dose of a shorter-acting stimulant to supplement if needed. You may elect to do this if the longer-acting morning stimulant fully controls symptoms, but wears off earlier than desired. Help set patient expectations that they will typically not be able to have symptom control for the entire day including evening. They should time their first daily dose to coincide with when they need to accomplish tasks, including getting ready to leave camp in the morning if needed.

As you may have noticed, many of the methylphenidate and amphetamine products have multiple brand names. At risk of causing further confusion, this paragraph attempts to explain the categorization of generic and brand name medications in Tables BB and CC. Methylphenidate and methylphenidate hydrochloride (HCl) are essentially the same medication without difference in effect. Branded methylphenidate is called Ritalin, whereas branded methylphenidate HCl is Metadate. Methylin, just to cause additional confusion, is a "branded generic of Ritalin" and is methylphenidate HCl. Dextroamphetamine brand names are Dexedrine and Dextrostat, but they are the same medication. Because the least expensive medication is typically the best option for street medicine, the differences in the brand names and dosage forms likely do not matter. Rarely, if ever, do street medicine patients request a specific generic such as dextroamphetamine rather than mixed amphetamine salts. Patients may tell you methamphetamine can be prescribed—and it can!—just not at the street doses most of your patients use.

4.8.1.3 Shortages of Prescription Stimulants

As of this handbook's publication, there is a shortage of most stimulant medications in North America. You may be able to substitute one similar generic for another in order for your patients to be able to have their medications. Many street medicine patients report being "treated like an addict," as in stigmatized or discriminated against, by some pharmacies when they are frustrated at being unable to obtain their prescription due to shortages. You can help your patient avoid this experience by calling several pharmacies in advance of sending the prescription to determine which generics, which doses, and how many pills they have in stock. Stable patients who do not need to be seen every month for their ADHD medication will need to have separate prescriptions sent into U.S. pharmacies for each 30-day supply, as refills are not allowed for stimulant prescriptions. Many prescribers send a two- or three-month supply of medications by sending two to three separate prescriptions for the same medication—this practice is common and expected by pharmacists.

4.8.1.4 Stimulant Side Effects

The most common adverse effects of stimulants are reduced appetite, headache, and insomnia. Tachycardia, elevated blood pressure, dizziness, gastrointestinal distress, dry mouth, and anxiety may also occur. People with preexisting anxiety may, however, experience some reduction in anxiety with ADHD treatment because it improves their ability to complete tasks and become organized. Other mental health diagnoses, such as psychotic disorders, bipolar disorder and tic disorders, can also worsen with stimulant use. Depression may improve with stimulants, as they are used as an adjunctive treatment for treatment-resistant depression. People with ADHD are at higher risk of epilepsy and vice versa, regardless of medication use. Stimulant medications for ADHD have not been associated with an increased risk of seizures or hospitalizations for seizures [99, 100].

4.8.2 Non-stimulant Medications for ADHD

Non-stimulant medications are considered second- and third-line treatments for adult ADHD after stimulants. Some patients may not be able to tolerate stimulants or you may determine that the risk of stimulants, given a patient's comorbidities, is too high. There are several options for non-stimulants, though they are typically less efficacious in adults than stimulants. Atomoxetine (Strattera), a second-line ADHD treatment, is a norepinephrine reuptake inhibitor that has better efficacy compared to non-stimulants in adults and has a better safety profile for the streets. Viloxazine extended-release (Qelbree), a more recently FDA-approved norepinephrine reuptake inhibitor, may have equal or better efficacy than atomoxetine, though there is no generic available in the United States [101]. Viloxazine ER is not yet approved in Canada. Other medications include short- and long-acting clonidine (Catapres, Kapvay), short- and long-acting guanfacine (Tenex, Intuniv), and bupropion XL (Wellbutrin XL) are third-line options for ADHD in adults. Neither guanfacine nor clonidine are ideal for street medicine due to the risk of rebound hypertension, with the possible exception of the clonidine transdermal patch (Catapres-TTS). Rarely, tricyclic antidepressants are used to treat ADHD, but are not recommended in the street medicine setting for reasons explained in the antidepressant section of this chapter. Bupropion XL carries the risk of seizures and is risky among street medicine patients for this reason.

4.8.2.1 Non-stimulant Dosing

Atomoxetine (Strattera) may be given once daily or divided in to two daily doses, once in the morning and once in the late afternoon. Viloxazine ER (Qelbree) is dosed once daily in the morning. Clonidine transdermal patches (Catapres-TTS) can be applied once weekly by a street medicine team member and need to be applied to an area of clean, hairless skin. Other formulations of clonidine are dosed two to three times per day and guanfacine (Tenex, Intuiv) is dosed nightly at bedtime. Dosing information for these non-stimulant medications is listed in Table 4.14.

4.8.2.2 Non-stimulant Side Effects

Atomoxetine (Strattera) and viloxazine ER (Qelbree), as norepinephrine reuptake inhibitors have similar side effects as other antidepressants in this class such as

Table 4.14 Dosing for non-stimulant medications for ADHD

Medication	Starting dose	Next dose	Next dose	Max dose	Other
Atomoxetine (Strattera)	40 mg Qam	80 mg Qam	100 mg Qam	100 mg Qam	Can be increased Q3 days
Bupropion XL (Wellbutrin XL)	150 mg Qam	300 mg Qam	450 mg Qam	450 mg Qam	Can be increased Q7 days
Clonidine tablets (Catapres)	0.1 mg Qhs	0.1 mg BID	0.1 mg Qam + 0.2 mg Qhs or 0.1 mg TID	0.2 mg BID	Not recommended for street medicine due to concern for rebound hypertension
Clonidine transdermal patch (Catapres-TTS)	0.1 mg/24 h applied Q7 days	0.2 mg/24 h applied Q7 days	0.3 mg/24 h applied Q7 days	0.3 mg/24 h applied Q7 days	Preferred for street medicine if clonidine is necessary. Increase Q7 days
Long-acting clonidine tablet (Kapvay)	0.1 mg Qhs	0.1 mg BID	0.1 mg Qam + 0.2 mg Qhs	0.2 mg BID	Use with caution on the streets due to rebound hypertension with abrupt discontinuation
Guanfacine immediate-release (Tenex)	1 mg Qhs	2 mg Qhs	3 mg Qhs	3 mg Qhs	May increase dose every 3–4 weeks. Risk of rebound hypertension is less than that for immediate release clonidine
Long-acting guanfacine (Intuniv)	1 mg Qhs	2 mg Qhs	3 mg Qhs	7 mg Qhs	Can increase dose every 3–4 weeks
Viloxazine ER (Qelbree)	200 mg Qam	400 mg Qam	600 mg Qam	600 mg Qam	Dose can be increased once weekly

venlafaxine (Effexor) and duloxetine (Cymbalta). They both have the FDA black box warning for an increase in suicidal thoughts in people younger than 25. Decreased appetite, upset stomach, nausea, vomiting, fatigue, insomnia, dizziness, tachycardia, and elevated blood pressure may also occur with atomoxetine and viloxazine. Taking these medications with food may reduce their GI side effects. While atomoxetine and viloxazine ER do not appear to cause significant discontinuation syndrome, patients can have GI symptoms and brain fog [102].

Guanfacine and clonidine products are both alpha agonists and may reduce blood pressure. Side effects include sedation, headaches, fatigue, stomach aches, nausea, dizziness, irritability, low blood pressure, mildly reduced appetite, and sexual side effects such as erectile dysfunction. Both can cause rebound hypertension with missed doses or abrupt cessation, with clonidine being worse than guanfacine. The clonidine transdermal patch is likely to be less problematic for rebound hypertension, particularly if the team can find the patient and replace the patch once weekly.

4.8.3 Other Treatments for ADHD

There is some mixed evidence related to cognitive behavioral therapy (CBT) for ADHD. Some studies noted it can be helpful combined with medication and even in the absence of medication treatment for ADHD [103]. However, given the effectiveness of stimulants and non-stimulants, CBT alone (without medication) is a fourth-line option after medication trials have failed or if the patient only wants CBT. CBT can be more helpful in navigating relationship challenges and interpersonal conflict that can occur with ADHD. See Chap. 11 for more information about CBT and other psychosocial interventions.

Occupational therapy (OT) for adults with ADHD, focused on improving practical and purposeful activities that allow people to live independently, can be helpful particularly in developing habits and routines to manage disorganization and improve executive function [104]. Even without a therapist or OT on the street medicine, any team member can assist patients with ADHD, by helping the person develop a routine for taking medications and structuring the day. They can assist with tracking appointments and other responsibilities on a calendar as well as setting phone or other alarm reminders. Whenever a street medicine team member provides the patient with instructions or information about medications and appointments, the team member should make sure to have the person's full attention for the best chance that the person will remember and be able to carry out instructions. If the person can read, written reminders are also helpful for forgetfulness and reinforcement.

References

1. Medication-Induced Dystonic Reactions Clinical Presentation: History, Physical Examination [Internet]. [cited 2025 May 11]. Available from: https://emedicine.medscape.com/article/814632-clinical
2. Lin D, Pilon D, Morrison L, Shah A, Lafeuille MH, Lefebvre P, et al. A cross-sectional study of patient out-of-pocket costs for antipsychotics among Medicaid beneficiaries with schizophrenia. Drugs Real World Outcomes [Internet]. 2023 Sep 1 [cited 2025 May 11];10(3):471. Available from: https://pmc.ncbi.nlm.nih.gov/articles/PMC10491554/
3. National Council for Mental Wellbeing. Guide to long-acting medications for clinicians and organizations. [Internet] [cited 2025 May 12].
4. Texas Health and Human Services. Long-acting injectable (LAI) antipsychotic quick reference chart. [Internet] 2024 Oct [cited 2025 Sept 25]. Available from: https://www.hhs.texas.gov/sites/default/files/documents/lai-antipsychotic-quick-reference.pdf
5. Aristada [package insert] Waltham, MA: Alkermes Inc; 2025. [cited 2025 May 12] Available from: https://www.accessdata.fda.gov/drugsatfda_docs/label/2025/207533s031lbl.pdf
6. Rykindo [package insert] Yantai, Shandong, China: Shandong Luye Pharmaceutical Company Ltd; 2025 [cited 2025 May 12] Available from: https://www.accessdata.fda.gov/drugsatfda_docs/label/2025/212849s001lbl.pdf

7. Huhn M, Nikolakopoulou A, Schneider-Thoma J, Krause M, Samara M, Peter N, et al. Comparative efficacy and tolerability of 32 oral antipsychotics for the acute treatment of adults with multi-episode schizophrenia: a systematic review and network meta-analysis. The Lancet [Internet]. 2019 Sep 14 [cited 2025 May 11];394(10202):939–51. Available from: https://www.thelancet.com/action/showFullText?pii=S0140673619311353
8. Atypical Antipsychotics May Be Safer Than Haloperidol for Delirium in MI Patients. NEJM Journal Watch [Internet]. 2018 Mar 29 [cited 2025 May 11];2018. Available from: https://www.jwatch.org/FW114015/2018/03/29/atypical-antipsychotics-may-be-safer-haloperidol-delirium
9. Leucht S, Cipriani A, Spineli L, Mavridis D, Örey D, Richter F, et al. Comparative efficacy and tolerability of 15 antipsychotic drugs in schizophrenia: A multiple-treatments meta-analysis. The Lancet [Internet]. 2013 [cited 2025 May 11];382(9896):951–962. Available from: https://pubmed.ncbi.nlm.nih.gov/23810019/
10. Kaul I, Sawchak S, Walling DP, Tamminga CA, Breier A, Zhu H, et al. Efficacy and safety of Xanomeline-Trospium Chloride in schizophrenia: a randomized clinical trial. JAMA Psychiatry [Internet]. 2024 Aug 1 [cited 2025 May 11];81(8):749–56. Available from: https://jamanetwork.com/journals/jamapsychiatry/fullarticle/2818047
11. Laszlovszky I, Barabássy Á, Németh G. Cariprazine, A Broad-Spectrum Antipsychotic for the Treatment of Schizophrenia: Pharmacology, Efficacy, and Safety. Adv Ther [Internet]. 2021 Jul 1 [cited 2025 May 11];38(7):3652. Available from: https://pmc.ncbi.nlm.nih.gov/articles/PMC8279990/
12. Sankaranarayanan A, Kazi S, Andrade C. Prevalence and predictors of QTc prolongation in patients seen in a clozapine clinic in a real-world setting in Australia. Schizophr Res [Internet]. 2024 Jun 1 [cited 2025 May 11];268:145–9. Available from: https://www.sciencedirect.com/science/article/abs/pii/S0920996423003432?via%3Dihub
13. Rummel-Kluge C, Komossa K, Schwarz S, Hunger H, Schmid F, Lobos CA, et al. Head-to-head comparisons of metabolic side effects of second generation antipsychotics in the treatment of schizophrenia: a systematic review and meta-analysis. Schizophr Res [Internet]. 2010 Nov [cited 2025 May 11];123(2–3):225. Available from: https://pmc.ncbi.nlm.nih.gov/articles/PMC2957510/
14. Dayabandara M, Hanwella R, Ratnatunga S, Seneviratne S, Suraweera C, de Silva VA. Antipsychotic-associated weight gain: management strategies and impact on treatment adherence. Neuropsychiatr Dis Treat [Internet]. 2017 Aug 22 [cited 2025 May 11];13:2231. Available from: https://pmc.ncbi.nlm.nih.gov/articles/PMC5574691/
15. Tsai J, Rosenheck RA. Obesity among chronically homeless adults: is it a problem? Public Health Rep [Internet]. 2013 [cited 2025 May 11];128(1):29. Available from: https://pmc.ncbi.nlm.nih.gov/articles/PMC3514718/
16. Koh KA, Hoy JS, O'Connell JJ, Montgomery P. The Hunger–obesity paradox: obesity in the homeless. J Urban Health [Internet]. 2012 Dec [cited 2025 May 11];89(6):952. Available from: https://pmc.ncbi.nlm.nih.gov/articles/PMC3531350/
17. Ra CK, Hébert ET, Alexander A, Kendzor DE, Suchting R, Businelle MS. Unsheltered homeless and unstably housed adults have higher levels of stress and more health risk factors than sheltered homeless adults. J Soc Distress Homeless [Internet]. 2021 Jan 2 [cited 2025 May 11];32(1):42. Available from: https://pmc.ncbi.nlm.nih.gov/articles/PMC10281693/
18. Fitzgerald I, O'Connell J, Keating D, Hynes C, McWilliams S, Crowley EK. Metformin in the management of antipsychotic-induced weight gain in adults with psychosis: development of the first evidence-based guideline using GRADE methodology. Evid Based Ment Health [Internet]. 2021 Feb 1 [cited 2025 May 11];25(1):15. Available from: https://pmc.ncbi.nlm.nih.gov/articles/PMC8788031/
19. Duma SR, Fung VSC. Drug-induced movement disorders. Aust Prescr [Internet]. 2019 Apr 1 [cited 2025 May 11];42(2):56. Available from: https://pmc.ncbi.nlm.nih.gov/articles/PMC6478951/
20. Albert N, Catthoor K, Morrens M. Akathisia after chronic usage of synthetic cathinones: a case study. Front Psychiatry. 2022;13:1046486.

21. Kim DD, Procyshyn RM, Jones AA, Lee LHN, Panenka WJ, Stubbs JL, et al. Movement disorders associated with substance use in adults living in precarious housing or homelessness. Prog Neuropsychopharmacol Biol Psychiatry [Internet]. 2023 Aug 30 [cited 2025 May 11];126:110795. Available from: https://www.sciencedirect.com/science/article/abs/pii/S0278584623000817
22. Harten PN van, Hoek HW, Kahn RS. Acute dystonia induced by drug treatment. BMJ: Br Med J [Internet]. 1999 Sep 4 [cited 2025 May 11];319(7210):623. Available from: https://pmc.ncbi.nlm.nih.gov/articles/PMC1116493/
23. Loonen AJM, Ivanova SA. Neurobiological mechanisms associated with antipsychotic drug-induced dystonia. J Psychopharmacol [Internet]. 2020 Jan 1 [cited 2025 May 11];35(1):3. Available from: https://pmc.ncbi.nlm.nih.gov/articles/PMC7770213/
24. Caroff SN, Hurford I, Lybrand J, Campbell EC. Movement disorders induced by antipsychotic drugs: implications of the CATIE Schizophrenia Trial. Neurol Clin [Internet]. 2011 Feb [cited 2025 May 11];29(1):127. Available from: https://pmc.ncbi.nlm.nih.gov/articles/PMC3018852/
25. van Harten PN, Hoek HW, Kahn RS. Acute dystonia induced by drug treatment. BMJ: Br Med J [Internet]. 1999 Sep 4 [cited 2025 May 11];319(7210):623. Available from: https://pmc.ncbi.nlm.nih.gov/articles/PMC1116493/
26. Kalniunas A, Chakrabarti I, Mandalia R, Munjiza J, Pappa S. The relationship between antipsychotic-induced akathisia and suicidal behaviour: a systematic review. Neuropsychiatr Dis Treat [Internet]. 2021 [cited 2025 May 11];17:3489–97. Available from: https://www.tandfonline.com/doi/pdf/10.2147/NDT.S337785
27. Wu H, Siafis S, Wang D, Burschinski A, Schneider-Thoma J, Priller J, et al. Antipsychotic-induced akathisia in adults with acute schizophrenia: a systematic review and dose-response meta-analysis. Eur Neuropsychopharmacol [Internet]. 2023 Jul 1 [cited 2025 May 11];72:40–9. Available from: https://www.sciencedirect.com/science/article/abs/pii/S0924977X23000664?via%3Dihub
28. Gerolymos C, Barazer R, Yon DK, Loundou A, Boyer L, Fond G. Drug efficacy in the treatment of antipsychotic-induced akathisia: a systematic review and network meta-analysis. JAMA Netw Open [Internet]. 2024 Mar 4 [cited 2025 May 11];7(3):e241527–e241527. Available from: https://jamanetwork.com/journals/jamanetworkopen/fullarticle/2815790
29. Berman BD. Neuroleptic malignant syndrome: a review for neurohospitalists. Neurohospitalist [Internet]. 2011 [cited 2025 May 11];1(1):41. Available from: https://pmc.ncbi.nlm.nih.gov/articles/PMC3726098/
30. Racz R, Soldatos TG, Jackson D, Burkhart K. Association between serotonin syndrome and second-generation antipsychotics via pharmacological target-adverse event analysis. Clin Transl Sci [Internet]. 2018 May 1 [cited 2025 May 11];11(3):322. Available from: https://pmc.ncbi.nlm.nih.gov/articles/PMC5944571/
31. Scotton WJ, Hill LJ, Williams AC, Barnes NM. Serotonin syndrome: pathophysiology, clinical features, management, and potential future directions. Int J Tryptophan Res [Internet]. 2019 [cited 2025 May 11];12:1178646919873925. Available from: https://pmc.ncbi.nlm.nih.gov/articles/PMC6734608/
32. Huang MW, Gibson RC, Jayaram MB, Caroff SN. Antipsychotics for schizophrenia spectrum disorders with catatonic symptoms. Cochrane Database Syst Rev [Internet]. 2022 Jul 12 [cited 2025 May 11];2022(7):CD013100. Available from: https://pmc.ncbi.nlm.nih.gov/articles/PMC9289703/
33. Beach S, Francis A, Fricchione G. Neuropsychiatry of Catatonia: Clinical Implications [Internet]. Psychiatric Times. 2019 [cited 2025 Sept 25]. Available from: https://www.psychiatrictimes.com/view/neuropsychiatry-catatonia-clinical-implications
34. Park YW, Kim Y, Lee JH. Antipsychotic-induced sexual dysfunction and its management. World J Mens Health [Internet]. 2012 [cited 2025 May 11];30(3):153. Available from: https://pmc.ncbi.nlm.nih.gov/articles/PMC3623530/
35. Balon R. Medications and sexual function and dysfunction. [Internet]. 2009 Oct [cited 2025 May 11];7(4):481–90. Available from: https://doi.org/101176/foc74.foc481

36. Montejo AL. Prolactin awareness: an essential consideration for physical health in schizophrenia. Eur Neuropsychopharmacol [Internet]. 2008 [cited 2025 May 11];18(SUPPL. 2):S108–14. Available from: https://pubmed.ncbi.nlm.nih.gov/18346598/
37. Johnson & Johnson has to pay $8 billion after male breast growth linked to antipsychotic drug | CNN [Internet]. [cited 2025 May 11]. Available from: https://www.cnn.com/2019/10/09/uk/johnson-and-johnson-male-breast-growth-damages/index.html
38. Chen JX, Su YA, Bian QT, Wei LH, Zhang RZ, Liu YH, et al. Adjunctive aripiprazole in the treatment of risperidone-induced hyperprolactinemia: a randomized, double-blind, placebo-controlled, dose-response study. Psychoneuroendocrinology [Internet]. 2015 Aug 1 [cited 2025 May 11];58:130–40. Available from: https://pubmed.ncbi.nlm.nih.gov/25981348/
39. Hwang T, Shah T, Sadeghi-Nejad H. A review of antipsychotics and priapism. Sex Med Rev [Internet]. 2021 Jul 1 [cited 2025 May 11];9(3):464–71. Available from: https://www.sciencedirect.com/science/article/abs/pii/S2050052120301128
40. Gottsch HP, Berger RE, Yang CC. Priapism: comorbid factors and treatment outcomes in a contemporary series. Adv Urol [Internet]. 2012 [cited 2025 May 11];2012:672624. Available from: https://pmc.ncbi.nlm.nih.gov/articles/PMC3395114/
41. Weiner DM, Lowe FC. Psychotropic drug-induced priapism: incidence, mechanism and management. CNS Drugs. 1998;9(5):371–9.
42. Druschky K, Bleich S, Grohmann R, Engel RR, Neyazi A, Stübner S, et al. Seizure rates under treatment with antipsychotic drugs: data from the AMSP project. World J Biol Psychiatry [Internet]. 2019 Oct 21 [cited 2025 May 11];20(9):732–41. Available from: https://pubmed.ncbi.nlm.nih.gov/30058414/
43. Górska N, Słupski J, Cubała WJ. Antipsychotic drugs in epilepsy. Neurol Neurochir Pol [Internet]. 2019 Dec 31 [cited 2025 May 11];53(6):408–12. Available from: https://pubmed.ncbi.nlm.nih.gov/31681966/
44. Berling I, Buckley NA, Isbister GK. The antipsychotic story: changes in prescriptions and overdose without better safety. Br J Clin Pharmacol [Internet]. 2016 [cited 2025 May 11];82(1):249. Available from: https://pmc.ncbi.nlm.nih.gov/articles/PMC4917785/
45. Nelson JC, Spyker DA. Morbidity and mortality associated with medications used in the treatment of depression: an analysis of cases reported to U.S. poison control centers, 2000–2014. Am J Psychiatry [Internet]. 2017 May 1 [cited 2025 May 11];174(5):438–50. Available from: https://doi.org/10.1176/appi.ajp.2016.16050523?
46. Zuschlag ZD. Second-generation antipsychotics and suicide: a commentary. J Clin Psychiatry. 2021;82(5)
47. Giambarberi L, Alexander HB, Clary HM. ADHD in adults with epilepsy: a guide for neurologists. Epilepsy Behav Rep [Internet]. 2025 Mar 1 [cited 2025 May 11];29:100739. Available from: https://www.sciencedirect.com/science/article/pii/S2589986424000960
48. Damegunta SR. Time matters!: when is the right time to estimate serum valproic acid levels? Indian J Psychol Med [Internet]. 2014 [cited 2025 May 11];36(3):349. Available from: https://pmc.ncbi.nlm.nih.gov/articles/PMC4100435/
49. Wang XQ, Xiong J, Xu WH, Yu SY, Huang XS, Zhang JT, et al. Risk of a lamotrigine-related skin rash: current meta-analysis and postmarketing cohort analysis. Seizure [Internet]. 2015 Feb 1 [cited 2025 May 11];25:52–61. Available from: https://www.seizure-journal.com/action/showFullText?pii=S1059131114003124
50. Farkas, Josh. Valproic acid intoxication – EMCrit Project [Internet]. 2024 June 29 [cited 2025 May 11]. Available from: https://emcrit.org/ibcc/vpa/
51. Patel AR, Nagalli S. Valproate toxicity. StatPearls [Internet]. 2024 May 6 [cited 2025 May 11]; Available from: https://www.ncbi.nlm.nih.gov/books/NBK560898/
52. Arnold PIM, Janzing JGE, Hommersom A. Machine learning for antidepressant treatment selection in depression. Drug Discov Today [Internet]. 2024 Aug 1 [cited 2025 May 10];29(8):104068. Available from: https://www.sciencedirect.com/science/article/pii/S1359644624001934
53. Depression Medication Choice Decision Aid [Internet]. [cited 2025 May 10]. Available from: https://depressiondecisionaid.mayoclinic.org/index

54. Browning M, Bilderbeck AC, Dias R, Dourish CT, Kingslake J, Deckert J, et al. The clinical effectiveness of using a predictive algorithm to guide antidepressant treatment in primary care (PReDicT): an open-label, randomised controlled trial. Neuropsychopharmacology [Internet]. 2021 Jun 1 [cited 2025 May 10];46(7):1307–14. Available from: https://www.nature.com/articles/s41386-021-00981-z
55. Trivedi MH, Rush AJ, Crismon ML, Kashner TM, Toprac MG, Carmody TJ, et al. Clinical results for patients with major depressive disorder in the Texas Medication Algorithm Project. Arch Gen Psychiatry [Internet]. 2004 Jul 1 [cited 2025 May 10];61(7):669–80. Available from: https://jamanetwork.com/journals/jamapsychiatry/fullarticle/482026
56. Pigott HE, Kim T, Xu C, Kirsch I, Amsterdam J. What are the treatment remission, response and extent of improvement rates after up to four trials of antidepressant therapies in real-world depressed patients? A reanalysis of the STAR*D study's patient-level data with fidelity to the original research protocol. BMJ Open [Internet]. 2023 Jul 25 [cited 2025 May 10];13(7). Available from: https://pubmed.ncbi.nlm.nih.gov/37491091/
57. Erickson BR, Ehrie J, Murray S, Dougherty RJ, Wainberg ML, Dixon LB, et al. A rapid review of 'low-threshold' psychiatric medication prescribing: considerations for street medicine and beyond. Psychiatr Serv [Internet]. 2022 Mar 1 [cited 2025 May 10];74(3):282. Available from: https://pmc.ncbi.nlm.nih.gov/articles/PMC9971341/
58. Table of Antidepressant Medications (Adults) [Internet]. [cited 2025 May 10]. Available from: https://ottawadepressionalgorithm.ca/en/content?id=38
59. Choosing an antidepressant for people with coronary heart disease – SPS – Specialist Pharmacy Service – The first stop for professional medicines advice [Internet]. [cited 2025 May 10]. Available from: https://www.sps.nhs.uk/articles/choosing-an-antidepressant-for-people-with-coronary-heart-disease/
60. Zwiebel SJ, Viguera AC. Discontinuing antidepressants: pearls and pitfalls. Cleve Clin J Med [Internet]. 2022 Jan 1 [cited 2025 May 10];89(1):18–26. Available from: https://www.ccjm.org/content/89/1/18
61. Allen R, Sharma U, Barlas S. Clinical experience with desvenlafaxine in treatment of pain associated with diabetic peripheral neuropathy. J Pain Res [Internet]. 2014 Jun 23 [cited 2025 May 10];7:339. Available from: https://pmc.ncbi.nlm.nih.gov/articles/PMC4075949/
62. Fortney JC, Unützer J, Wrenn G, Pyne JM, Smith GR, Schoenbaum M, et al. A tipping point for measurement-based care. Psychiatric Serv [Internet]. 2017 Feb 1 [cited 2025 May 10];68(2):179–88. Available from: https://doi.org/10.1176/appi.ps.201500439
63. Blevins CA, Weathers FW, Davis MT, Witte TK, Domino JL. The posttraumatic stress disorder checklist for DSM-5 (PCL-5): development and initial psychometric evaluation. J Trauma Stress. 2015;28(6):489–98.
64. Rea J. Social relationships, stigma, and wellbeing through experiences of homelessness in the United Kingdom. J Soc Issues [Internet]. 2023 Mar 1 [cited 2025 May 10];79(1):465–93. Available from: https://doi.org/10.1111/josi.12572
65. De Vries YA, Roest AM, Bos EH, Burgerhof JGM, Van Loo HM, De Jonge P. Predicting antidepressant response by monitoring early improvement of individual symptoms of depression: individual patient data meta-analysis. Br J Psychiatry [Internet]. 2018 Jan 1 [cited 2025 May 11];214(1):4. Available from: https://pmc.ncbi.nlm.nih.gov/articles/PMC7557872/
66. Henssler J, Alexander D, Schwarzer G, Bschor T, Baethge C. Combining antidepressants vs antidepressant monotherapy for treatment of patients with acute depression: a systematic review and meta-analysis. JAMA Psychiatry [Internet]. 2022 Apr 1 [cited 2025 May 11];79(4):300. Available from: https://pmc.ncbi.nlm.nih.gov/articles/PMC8851370/
67. Liu X, Momen NC, Molenaar N, Rommel AS, Bergink V, Munk-Olsen T. Discontinuation of antidepressants: is there a minimum time on treatment that will reduce relapse risk? J Affect Disord [Internet]. 2021 Jul 1 [cited 2025 May 11];290:254. Available from: https://pmc.ncbi.nlm.nih.gov/articles/PMC8739188/
68. Lye MS, Tey YY, Tor YS, Shahabudin AF, Ibrahimid N, Ling KH, et al. Predictors of recurrence of major depressive disorder. PLoS One [Internet]. 2020 [cited 2025 May 11];15(3):e0230363. Available from: https://pmc.ncbi.nlm.nih.gov/articles/PMC7082055/

69. Gelenberg AJ, Marlene Freeman CP, Markowitz JC, Rosenbaum JF, Thase ME, Trivedi MH, et al. Practice guideline for the treatment of patients with major depressive disorder third edition work group on major depressive disorder. 2010 [cited 2025 May 11]; Available from: http://www.psychiatryonline.com/pracGuide/pracGuideTopic_7.aspx.
70. Baldessarini RJ, Tondo L, Ghiani C, Lepri B. Illness risk following rapid versus gradual discontinuation of antidepressants. Am J Psychiatry [Internet]. 2010 Aug [cited 2025 May 11];167(8):934–41. Available from: https://doi.org/10.1176/appi.ajp.2010.09060880
71. Henssler J, Schmidt Y, Schmidt U, Schwarzer G, Bschor T, Baethge C. Incidence of antidepressant discontinuation symptoms: a systematic review and meta-analysis. Lancet Psychiatry [Internet]. 2024 Jul 1 [cited 2025 May 11];11(7):526–35. Available from: https://pubmed.ncbi.nlm.nih.gov/38851198/
72. Zhang MM, Tan X, Zheng YB, Zeng N, Li Z, Horowitz MA, et al. Incidence and risk factors of antidepressant withdrawal symptoms: a meta-analysis and systematic review. Mol Psychiatry [Internet]. 2024 May 1 [cited 2025 May 11];30(5). Available from: https://pubmed.ncbi.nlm.nih.gov/39394455/
73. Wilson E, Lader M. A review of the management of antidepressant discontinuation symptoms. Ther Adv Psychopharmacol [Internet]. 2015 [cited 2025 May 11];5(6):357. Available from: https://pmc.ncbi.nlm.nih.gov/articles/PMC4722507/
74. Davies J, Read J. A systematic review into the incidence, severity and duration of antidepressant withdrawal effects: are guidelines evidence-based? Addictive Behaviors [Internet]. 2019 Oct 1 [cited 2025 May 11];97:111–21. Available from: https://pubmed.ncbi.nlm.nih.gov/30292574/
75. Benazzi F. Fluoxetine for the treatment of SSRI discontinuation syndrome. Int J Neuropsychopharmacol [Internet]. 2008 Aug 1 [cited 2025 May 11];11(5):725–6. Available from: https://doi.org/10.1017/S1461145708008493
76. Hertfordshire Partnership University. Guidelines on choice and selection of antidepressants for the management of depression. [Internet] London, National Health Service, 2025 [cited 2025 May 11]. 25 p. Available from: https://www.hpft.nhs.uk/media/azlh5shc/hpft-guidelines-on-choice-and-selection-of-antidepressants-for-the-management-of-depression-v20-final-feb-2025.pdf
77. Behlke LM, Lenze EJ, Carney RM. The cardiovascular effects of newer antidepressants in older adults and those with or at high risk for cardiovascular diseases. CNS Drugs [Internet]. 2020 Nov 1 [cited 2025 May 11];34(11):1133. Available from: https://pmc.ncbi.nlm.nih.gov/articles/PMC7666056/
78. Maguire MJ, Weston J, Singh J, Marson AG. Antidepressants for people with epilepsy and depression. Cochrane Database of Syst Rev. 2014;2014(12)
79. Cho H, Lee K, Wang SM, Lee H, Kim S, Kim TH, et al. Global burden of antidepressant-associated seizures from 1967 to 2023: a comparative analysis of the international pharmacovigilance database. J Affect Disord [Internet]. 2025 Jul 15 [cited 2025 May 11];381:215–23. Available from: https://www.sciencedirect.com/science/article/abs/pii/S0165032725005853
80. Jing E, Straw-Wilson K. Sexual dysfunction in selective serotonin reuptake inhibitors (SSRIs) and potential solutions: a narrative literature review. Ment Health Clin [Internet]. 2016 Jul 1 [cited 2025 May 11];6(4):191. Available from: https://pmc.ncbi.nlm.nih.gov/articles/PMC6007725/
81. Waldinger MD. Psychiatric disorders and sexual dysfunction. Handb Clin Neurol [Internet]. 2015 [cited 2025 May 11];130:469–89. Available from: https://pubmed.ncbi.nlm.nih.gov/26003261/
82. Taylor MJ, Rudkin L, Hawton K. Strategies for managing antidepressant-induced sexual dysfunction: systematic review of randomised controlled trials. J Affect Disord [Internet]. 2005 Nov [cited 2025 May 11];88(3):241–54. Available from: https://pubmed.ncbi.nlm.nih.gov/16162361/
83. Khashaba S, Bruce A, Krishan A, Ehsanullah S, Ndrika S, Khela A. The effect of phosphodiesterase-5-inhibitor on female sexual function: a systematic review and

meta-analysis. J Sex Med [Internet]. 2023 Jun 27 [cited 2025 May 11];20(Supplement_3). Available from: https://doi.org/10.1093/jsxmed/qdad068.015

84. American Psychiatric Association. Joint statement on federal concerns about psychotropic medication safety [Internet]. 2025 Mar 21 [cited 2025 May 11]. Available from: https://www.psychiatry.org/News-room/News-Releases/Joint-Statement-on-Federal-Concerns-About-Psychotr
85. Fornaro M, Anastasia A, Valchera A, Carano A, Orsolini L, Vellante F, et al. The FDA "Black Box" warning on antidepressant suicide risk in young adults: More harm than benefits? Front Psychiatry [Internet]. 2019 [cited 2025 May 11];10(May):294. Available from: https://pmc.ncbi.nlm.nih.gov/articles/PMC6510161/
86. Peterlin BL, Katsnelson MJ, Calhoun AH. The associations between migraine, unipolar psychiatric comorbidities, and stress-related disorders and the role of estrogen. Curr Pain Headache Rep [Internet]. 2009 [cited 2025 May 11];13(5):404. Available from: https://pmc.ncbi.nlm.nih.gov/articles/PMC3972495/
87. Migraine headache and obsessive-compulsive symptoms in a student sample [Internet]. [cited 2025 May 11]. Available from: https://psychiatry-psychopharmacology.com/en/migraine-headache-and-obsessive-compulsive-symptoms-in-a-student-sample-131831
88. Steinert T, Fröscher W. Epileptic Seizures under antidepressive drug treatment: systematic review. Pharmacopsychiatry [Internet]. 2018 Jul 1 [cited 2025 May 11];51(4):121–35. Available from: https://pubmed.ncbi.nlm.nih.gov/28850959/
89. Hill T, Coupland C, Morriss R, Arthur A, Moore M, Hippisley-Cox J. Antidepressant use and risk of epilepsy and seizures in people aged 20 to 64 years: Cohort study using a primary care database. BMC Psychiatry [Internet]. 2015 Dec 17 [cited 2025 May 11];15(1):1–13. Available from: https://bmcpsychiatry.biomedcentral.com/articles/10.1186/s12888-015-0701-9
90. McKean J, Watts H, Mokszycki R. Breakthrough seizures after starting vilazodone for depression. Pharmacotherapy J Hum Pharmacol Drug Therapy [Internet]. 2015 Mar 1 [cited 2025 May 11];35(3):e6–8. Available from: https://doi.org/10.1002/phar.1549
91. Brancati GE, Magnesa A, Acierno D, Carli M, De Rosa U, Froli A, et al. Current nonstimulant medications for adults with attention-deficit/hyperactivity disorder. Expert Rev Neurother [Internet]. 2024 [cited 2025 May 11];24(8):743–59. Available from: https://pubmed.ncbi.nlm.nih.gov/38915262/
92. The ASAM/AAAP Clinical Practice Guideline on the Management of Stimulant Use Disorder. J Addict Med [Internet]. 2024 May 1 [cited 2025 May 11];18(1):1–56. Available from: https://journals.lww.com/journaladdictionmedicine/fulltext/2024/05001/the_asam_aaap_clinical_practice_guideline_on_the.1.aspx
93. Peterson K, McDonagh MS, Fu R. Comparative benefits and harms of competing medications for adults with attention-deficit hyperactivity disorder: a systematic review and indirect comparison meta-analysis. Psychopharmacology (Berl) [Internet]. 2008 Mar [cited 2025 May 11];197(1):1–11. Available from: https://pubmed.ncbi.nlm.nih.gov/18026719/
94. Huss M, Duhan P, Gandhi P, Chen CW, Spannhuth C, Kumar V. Methylphenidate dose optimization for ADHD treatment: review of safety, efficacy, and clinical necessity. Neuropsychiatr Dis Treat [Internet]. 2017 Jul 4 [cited 2025 May 11];13:1741. Available from: https://pmc.ncbi.nlm.nih.gov/articles/PMC5505611/
95. Cortese S, Adamo N, Del Giovane C, Mohr-Jensen C, Hayes AJ, Carucci S, et al. Comparative efficacy and tolerability of medications for attention-deficit hyperactivity disorder in children, adolescents, and adults: a systematic review and network meta-analysis. Lancet Psychiatry [Internet]. 2018 Sep 1 [cited 2025 May 11];5(9):727. Available from: https://pmc.ncbi.nlm.nih.gov/articles/PMC6109107/
96. Stimulant Dosing Limits | CARLAT PUBLISHING [Internet]. [cited 2025 May 11]. Available from: https://www.thecarlatreport.com/articles/4464-stimulant-dosing-limits
97. How to Select a Stimulant for Adult ADHD | CARLAT PUBLISHING [Internet]. [cited 2025 May 11]. Available from: https://www.thecarlatreport.com/articles/5341-how-to-select-a-stimulant-for-adult-adhd

98. Goodman DW. Lisdexamfetamine Dimesylate (Vyvanse), a prodrug stimulant for attention-deficit/hyperactivity disorder. Pharmacy and Therapeutics [Internet]. 2010 May [cited 2025 May 11];35(5):273. Available from: https://pmc.ncbi.nlm.nih.gov/articles/PMC2873712/
99. Liu X, Carney PR, Bussing R, Segal R, Cottler LB, Winterstein AG. Stimulants do not increase the risk of seizure-related hospitalizations in children with epilepsy. J Child Adolesc Psychopharmacol [Internet]. 2018 Mar 1 [cited 2025 May 11];28(2):111–6. Available from: https://doi.org/10.1089/cap.2017.0110?
100. Wiggs KK, Chang Z, Quinn PD, Hur K, Gibbons R, Dunn D, et al. Attention-deficit/hyperactivity disorder medication and seizures. Neurology. 2018;90(13):e1104–10.
101. Yu CL, Kao YC, Thompson T, Stubbs B, Tseng PT, Hsu CW, et al. Response trajectories and temporal trends of viloxazine treatment for young people with ADHD: a meta-analysis. JAMA Netw Open [Internet]. 2024 Nov 4 [cited 2025 May 11];7(11):e2445885–e2445885. Available from: https://jamanetwork.com/journals/jamanetworkopen/fullarticle/2826361
102. Robinson CL, Parker K, Kataria S, Downs E, Supra R, Kaye AD, et al. Viloxazine for the treatment of attention deficit hyperactivity disorder. Health Psychol Res [Internet]. 2022 [cited 2025 May 11];10(3):38360. Available from: https://pmc.ncbi.nlm.nih.gov/articles/PMC9501833/
103. Young Z, Moghaddam N, Tickle A. The efficacy of cognitive behavioral therapy for adults with ADHD: a systematic review and meta-analysis of randomized controlled trials. J Atten Disord [Internet]. 2020 Apr 1 [cited 2025 May 11];24(6):875–88. Available from: https://doi.org/10.1177/1087054716664413
104. Adamou M, Asherson P, Arif M, Buckenham L, Cubbin S, Dancza K, et al. Recommendations for occupational therapy interventions for adults with ADHD: a consensus statement from the UK adult ADHD network. BMC Psychiatry [Internet]. 2021 Dec 1 [cited 2025 May 11];21(1):72. Available from: https://pmc.ncbi.nlm.nih.gov/articles/PMC7863422/

5 Substance Use: Assessment and Guiding Principles for Street Medicine

5.1 Introduction

Substance use is common among people living unsheltered, often as a means of survival. Unsheltered individuals report using substances (drugs and alcohol) to numb depression and anxiety symptoms or improve mood, stay awake for self-protection, and to avoid loneliness [1]. In a 2023 study of street medicine teams in California, all respondents reported substance use disorder (SUD) diagnoses among at least 20% of patients and three-quarters reported SUD among more than 50% of patients [2]. California policy lab compared self-report of people who are homeless, with 75% of unsheltered and 13% sheltered individuals reporting substance use disorders [3]. Comorbid mental health and substance use disorders are more common among people living unsheltered than people living in homeless shelters as is tri-morbidity, defined as having a physical, mental, and substance use diagnosis [3, 4]. Substance use disorders contribute substantially to disproportionate deaths between unsheltered, sheltered, and housed adults. During a 10-year prospective study, unsheltered adults were 46 times more likely to die from a substance use disorder than the general population and 2.5 times more likely to die than adults living in shelters [5].

People who are homeless report receiving substandard care due to stigma and discrimination when seeking help for mental health, substance use, and chronic pain and report being made to feel inhuman and unwelcome in healthcare settings [6, 7]. Hoffman and Coffey explain that similar experiences with providers of homeless social services cause homeless individuals to feel objectified (treated as a number) and infantilized, resulting in a withdrawal of service in order to "maintain a sense of dignity and self-respect." [8] These concepts resonate with street medicine clinicians who observe their unsheltered patients avoiding mainstream healthcare at all cost, especially when the health issue related substance use. To avoid repeating these mistakes, street medicine teams focus on providing care that is patient-led, reality-based, and demonstrates unconditional respect [9].

S. Hatcher et al., *Street Mental Health Handbook*,
https://doi.org/10.1007/978-3-032-00663-9_5

5.2 Interviews with Street Medicine Clinicians

For assistance with this chapter and Chap. 6, I informally interviewed street medicine clinicians working in the United States (U.S.) who I know through work with the Street Medicine Institute or who were recommended to me as experts in street-based addiction medicine. My coauthors shared information about common interventions and practices in Canada and their experiences working in street medicine in Ottawa. There are very few publications related to treating and preventing harm from problematic substance use in the street medicine setting or that focus primarily on interventions for people sleeping rough. These informal interviews with street medicine clinicians were not intended as scientific research and do not meet criteria for it. Rather, during the interviews, I attempted to gather information on what and how street medicine clinicians are doing, despite the paucity of research, to care for people sleeping rough with incredibly complex physical, mental, and substance use disorders. I present information from my interviews, my own practices, and information from research about substance use treatment in the street medicine setting as well as research on substance use and interventions in various unsheltered, sheltered, and housed populations where available. I was impressed with how much variability exists from city to city—even within neighborhoods—in commonly used drugs, contamination in the drug supply, community resource availability, policies and laws that impact people using drugs, and what capacity different street medicine teams have to implement interventions. From my perspective, the only clear gold-standard practices for problematic substance use in the street medicine setting are harm reduction, letting our patients take the lead and set the goals, and willingness to accompany people on their journeys whatever choices they make. Hopefully, you will find the information in this chapter and the next chapter useful in weighing the risks and benefits of various treatment options, considering how to tailor interventions for the streets, and determining what practices align with your team's values and risk tolerance in the unique setting where you work.

5.3 Letting the Patient Take the Lead

One of the core concepts of the street medicine is to "go to the people." According to the Street Medicine Institute, going to the people includes not only providing health and social services for people living unsheltered in their own environment but also meeting people on their own terms [10]. People who are homeless and use drugs have expressed in qualitative research a preference for approaches to substance use treatment that value their autonomy and priorities over abstinence [11]. Desired qualities of service providers include empathy, person-centeredness, humility, acceptance, and respect for their autonomy [12]. Consistency in the relationship and knowing the service provider was there for them helps people who are homeless feel better and less alone [13].

5.4 Harm Reduction

Traditional approaches to substance use have often prioritized abstinence-based interventions and punitive criminal justice responses. However, in recent decades, harm reduction has emerged as an alternative strategy focused not necessarily on eliminating drug use, but on minimizing the adverse health, social, and legal impacts associated with it. Harm reduction is rooted in principles of human rights, pragmatism, and public health. Harm reduction refers to "policies, programs and practices that aim to reduce the harms associated with the use of psychoactive drugs in people unable or unwilling to stop using them" [14]. This approach recognizes drug use as a part of our world and emphasizes meeting people *where they are*, rather than demanding cessation. Abstinence is often not a goal for people sleeping rough.

Successful street medicine teams focus on creative methods to reduce harm both from drugs and having to use them in unsanitary environments. The photo below from street medicine rounds in Atlanta, Georgia, highlights the need for harm reduction and the reality that recovery is nearly impossible when sleeping outside. Harm reduction strategies include safer supply where legal, community naloxone distribution and education, distribution of clean needles and other safe-use gear, and safe consumption or safe observation facilities.

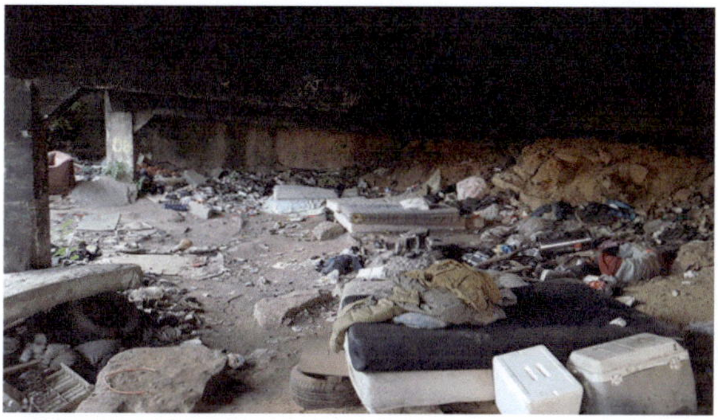

Photo credit: Liz Frye

5.4.1 Harm Reduction Policy

Globally, harm reduction has been embraced to varying degrees. Countries like Portugal, which decriminalized drug possession in 2001, have integrated harm reduction into a comprehensive public health strategy. This model has led to declines in drug-related deaths, HIV transmission, and incarceration rates [15]. Similarly, Switzerland's heroin-assisted treatment programs have demonstrated reduced crime and improved quality of life for participants [16]. In Canada, harm reduction is recognized as one of the four pillars of the national drug strategy. The proliferation of supervised consumption sites in British Columbia, for example, has been a direct response to the opioid overdose crisis. However, political shifts and legal restrictions continue to impede expansion in some provinces. Hard-won harm reduction policies in the U.S. have been plagued by roll-backs in recent years; Oregon ended its decriminalization of drug use in 2023.

5.4.2 Needle and Syringe Programs (NSPs)

These programs, also called syringe service providers (SSP), provide sterile injecting equipment to reduce soft tissue infections from unsanitary equipment and stop the transmission of blood-borne viruses such as HIV and hepatitis C caused by sharing supplies. A Cochrane review concluded that NSPs are associated with significant reductions in hepatitis C incidence among people who inject drugs [17]. Most programs also offer supplies of fentanyl and xylazine test strips. While test strips do not necessarily stop people from using their adulterated drugs, they do tend to engage in safer behaviors, such as not using alone, when they know the contents of their drugs.

5.4.3 Opioid Agonist Therapy (OAT)/Medications for Opioid Use Disorder (MOUD)

Treatments like methadone and buprenorphine reduce illicit opioid use, overdose risk, and criminal activity. OAT is also associated with better social functioning and reduced mortality [18].

5.4.4 Supervised Consumption Sites (SCS)

Also known as safe injection sites, SCS provide a medically supervised environment for drug use. Evidence from Vancouver's Insite program indicates reductions in fatal overdoses, increased referrals to treatment, and no increase in crime [19]. Supervised consumption sites often also run needle and syringe programs.

5.4.5 Naloxone Distribution

Widespread access to naloxone, an opioid overdose reversal agent, has saved thousands of lives and is increasingly endorsed by public health authorities [20]. The entire community needs access to naloxone—not just people who use drugs, harm reduction workers, or street outreach and street medicine teams—as community members often act as life guards for people sleeping rough in their neighborhoods or areas of work.

5.4.6 Safer Supply

Safer supply programs prescribe medications, usually opioids but sometimes stimulants, to people who are at high risk of overdose and also want to begin controlling their substance use. In safe opioid programs, clients are prescribed a long acting morphine, often morphine sulfate (Kadian) as well as hydromorphone (Dilaudid) which provides a high and helps to manage withdrawal and reduce cravings. Dispensing options include daily take-homes from a pharmacy or observed use in peer managed spaces. Safer supply, while legal in Canada, is currently illegal in the United States.

The benefits of these programs are that users are less exposed to the toxic drug supply that contains lethal contaminants such as xylazine or other synthetic opioids, which often result in overdose and death. Providing a safe supply reduces the risk of overdose and can start a conversation about stabilization and rehabilitation.

Many people who use drugs engage in survival-driven activities, such as petty theft or sex work, to fund their drug use; safer supply protects users from having to engage in risky, harmful activities. By providing a legal and free or low-cost alternative, safer supply reduces the financial burden of drug dependency. As a result, there is a decreased risk of incarceration linked to substance use, which can be both psychologically traumatizing as well as deadly when opioid users lose their tolerance. Safer supply eases pressure on the criminal justice system and improves community safety as well.

People sleeping rough are also able to spend less time and energy seeking drugs and focus more on their physical and mental health. Safer supply can act as a gateway to broader health and social supports. By stabilizing substance use and reducing the chaos associated with sourcing drugs, participants are more likely to access primary care, housing services, mental health support, and income assistance. This stabilization can improve overall health outcomes and foster trust in healthcare systems that many people distrust due to stigma and discrimination.

Unlike traditional abstinence-based models, safer supply respects the autonomy of individuals who are not ready or willing to stop using drugs. It offers a noncoercive, patient-centered model of care that meets people where they are. This approach can be lifesaving for individuals who have not succeeded with or declined medication for OUD and foster a sense of dignity and self-determination.

Safer supply programs have been criticized for several reasons: being a source of drugs on the street as people will "divert" or sell their safe supply to others, creating unintended consequences for the wider population of opioid users, and creating a risk to public safety. Diversion can pose a public health risk if diverted drugs are misused or fall into the hands of individuals with lower tolerances. Some critics argue that this could perpetuate drug dependency rather than reduce it.

While early qualitative and observational data are promising, there is a lack of robust, long-term, randomized controlled trials evaluating the effectiveness and cost-efficiency of safer supply programs. A scoping review on prescribed safer opioid supply found reductions in opioid overdoses, a reduction in street drug use, an increase in health system use, reduced infectious complications, and improvements in mental health [21]. Clients and providers identified insufficient opioid doses and a limited range of opioid options within safer opioid supply programs as potential factors contributing to diversion and hindering program access. A study from British Columbia of a large retrospective population-based cohort of opioid safe supply found a reduction in overdose related and all-cause mortality [22]. However, there are gaps in the evidence particularly long-term studies of efficacy, comparisons with other treatments for OUD and the prevalence and impact of diversion.

From a policy standpoint, safer supply programs raise questions about the role of the state in managing drug use although there are double standards if comparing opioid or stimulant regulation with alcohol. Alcohol users have supervised consumptions sites (bars) with safer supply and alcohol use is governed by regulation. A hundred years ago when prohibition was in place in the United States, the conversation was not dissimilar to that of the opioid epidemic now with widespread concern about illegal alcohol being tainted with toxins (often methanol) causing significant mortality and morbidity.

5.5 Trauma-Informed Substance Use Assessments

Substance use assessments, whether performed in the street medicine setting or not, should be extremely nonjudgmental, both for the sake of the relationship with your patient and for best approximations of substance use. Chapter 3, Making the Diagnosis, discussed some assessment for substance use, as it should be a part of a good mental health evaluation given the overlap between symptoms caused by substance use and other mental health diagnoses. When you're assessing substance use for helping someone to use less or quit, you will need to know more details than you would for the purposes of the Rapid Street Psych Assessment. Substance use history-taking should not be exhaustive for every drug or sip of alcohol a person has ever taken, unless you want your patient to avoid you in the future. See Fig. 5.1 for an example initial conversation about substance use between you (dashed line) and your friend, Sideways (solid line). Sideways uses they/them pronouns. Remember to ask permission to talk about substance use before you get started.

The conversation in Fig. 5.1 started an important conversation in which Sideways expressed concern about their drinking and indicated a desire to cut back or quit. Note that in this conversation, you focused on what Sideways wanted to do and did not push Sideways to cut back or quit fentanyl first or at the same time as trying to cut back or quit drinking. Even though we are concerned about how quickly an overdose on fentanyl could kill or harm our patients, we should not try to get someone to cut back or quit if they express not being ready, especially when they have already discussed the difficulty of changing drinking habits. Offering harm reduction supplies to reduce the negative consequences and overdose from fentanyl is a great step towards Sideways' goal of not dying from an overdose.

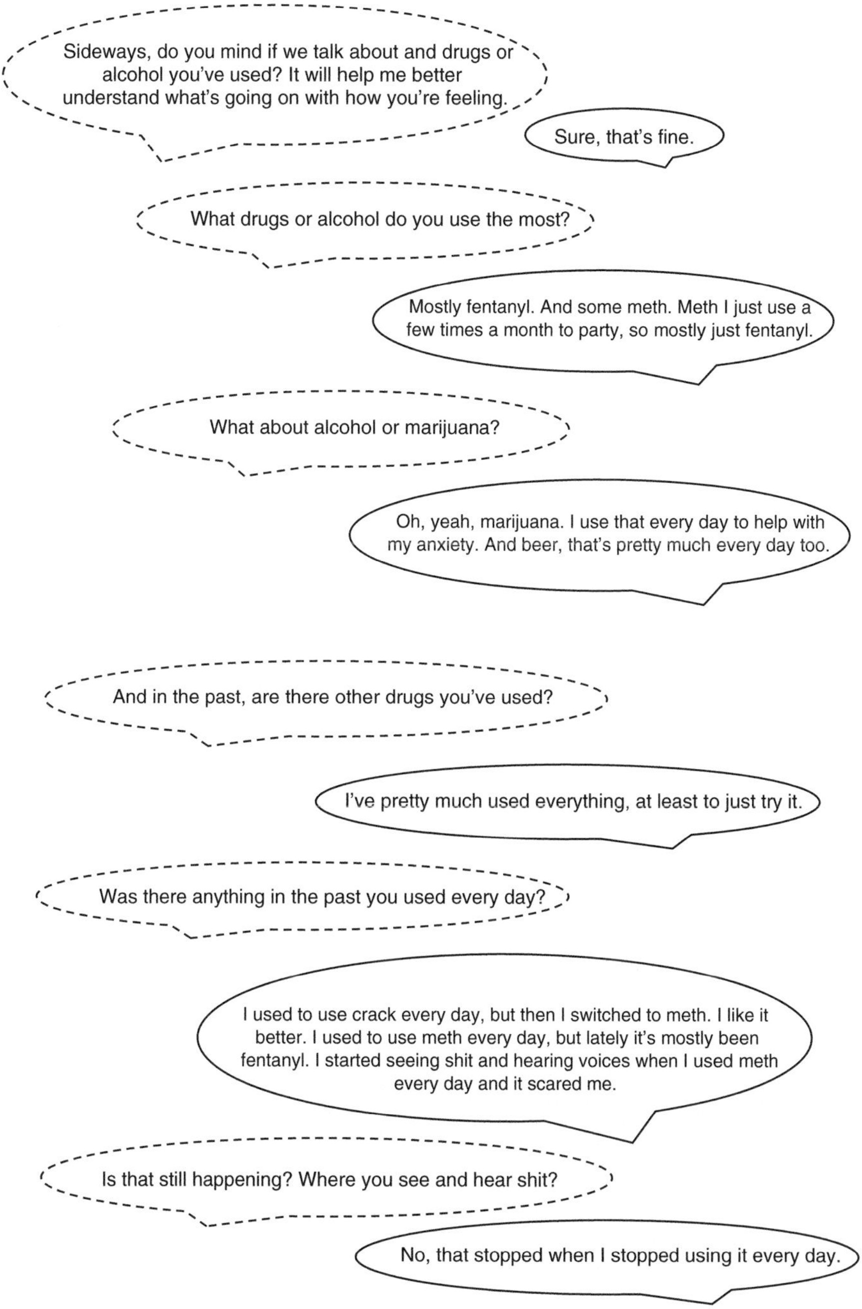
Sideways, do you mind if we talk about and drugs or alcohol you've used? It will help me better understand what's going on with how you're feeling.
Sure, that's fine.
What drugs or alcohol do you use the most?
Mostly fentanyl. And some meth. Meth I just use a few times a month to party, so mostly just fentanyl.
What about alcohol or marijuana?
Oh, yeah, marijuana. I use that every day to help with my anxiety. And beer, that's pretty much every day too.
And in the past, are there other drugs you've used?
I've pretty much used everything, at least to just try it.
Was there anything in the past you used every day?
I used to use crack every day, but then I switched to meth. I like it better. I used to use meth every day, but lately it's mostly been fentanyl. I started seeing shit and hearing voices when I used meth every day and it scared me.
Is that still happening? Where you see and hear shit?
No, that stopped when I stopped using it every day.

Fig. 5.1 Conversation with Sideways

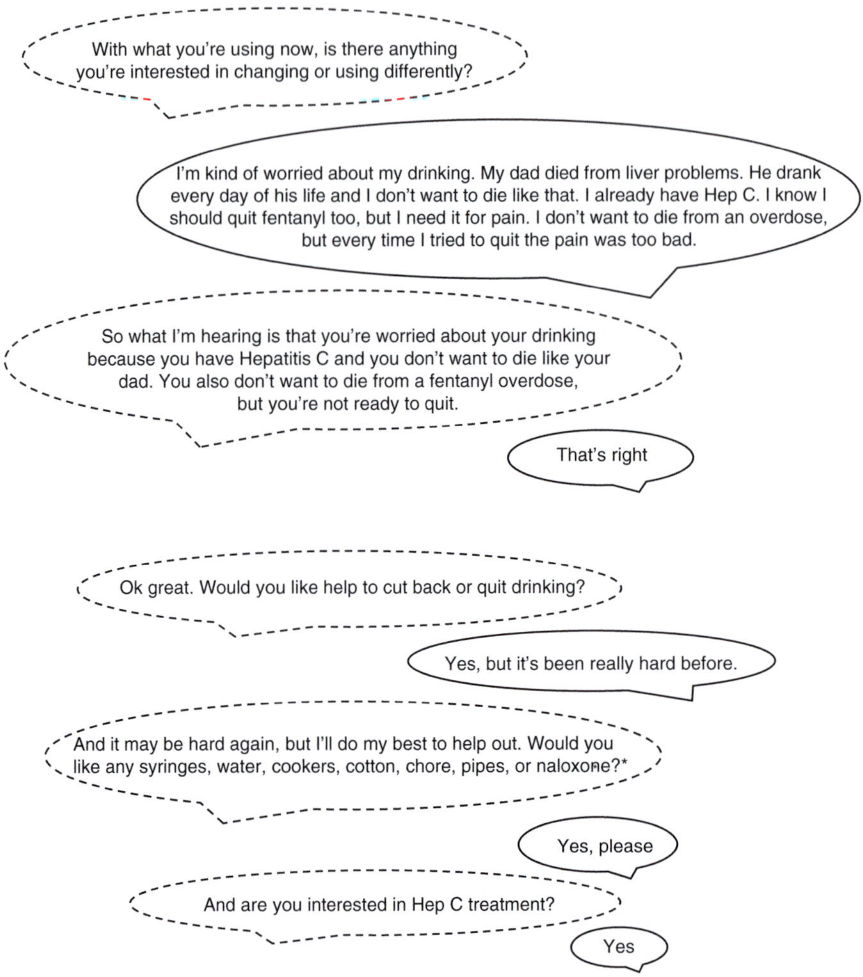

Fig. 5.1 (continued)

The next step in helping Sideways is to quantify how much and what kind of alcohol they drink. You will want to understand their level of tolerance and the likelihood that they will develop withdrawal symptoms. Knowing their patterns of alcohol use, how long their current episode of use has lasted, whether they have experienced withdrawal in the past, and what complications they had with past withdrawal will guide the plans Sideways and you make for treatment. Figure 5.2 is an example of this conversation with Sideways.

In addition to asking Sideways what they drink, how much, and how often, ask about withdrawal symptoms in the past including seizures and delirium tremens (DTs). Ask about times they've quit or tried to quit, how it went, what is the longest time they've quit, and what led to them drinking again. While this conversation with

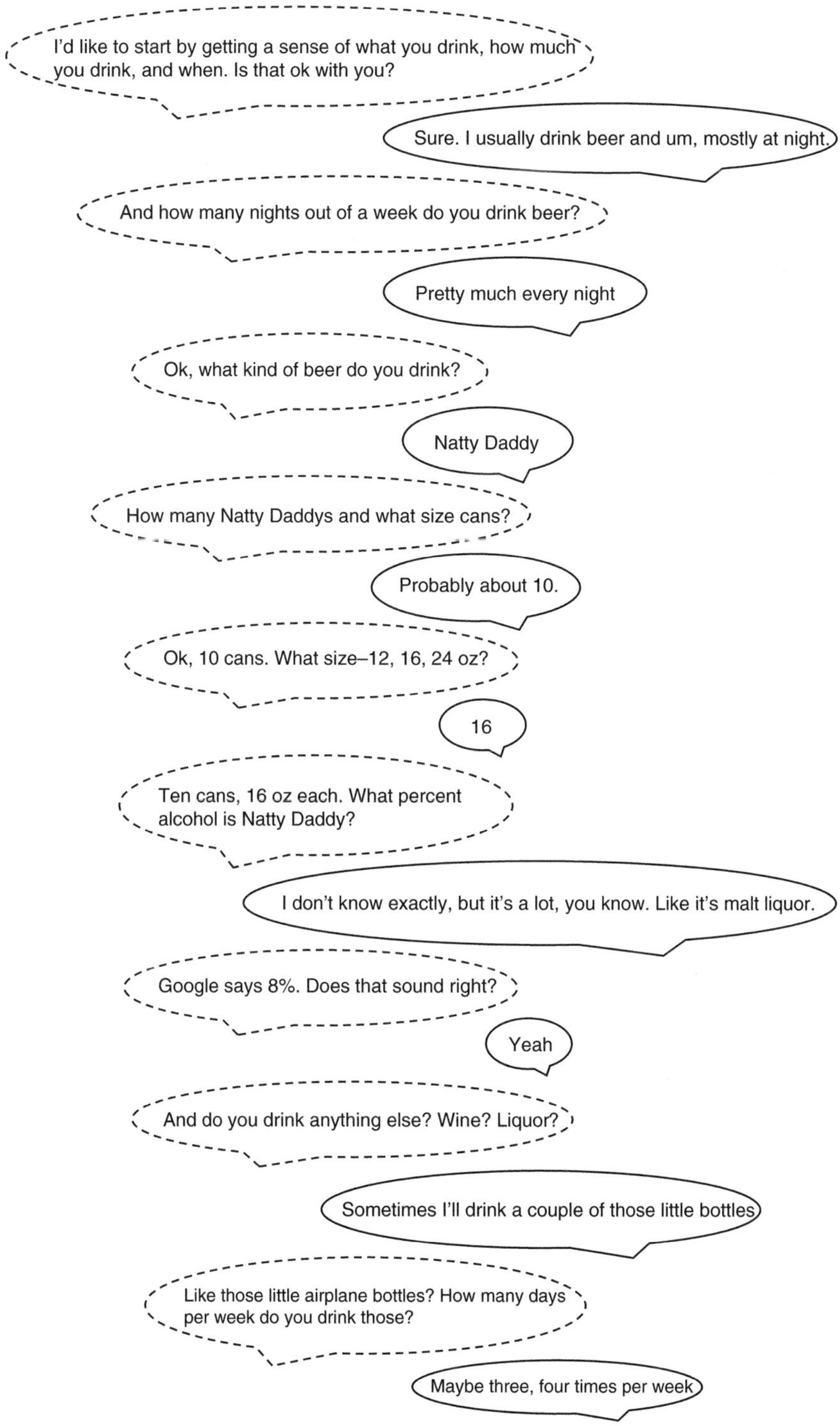

Fig. 5.2 Quantifying Sideways' Alcohol Use

Sideways is about alcohol, it serves as a guide for asking about other substances as well.

The next chapter in this handbook, Chap. 6, addresses the effects of substance use, health complications of substance use, harm reduction related to individual substances, as well as available treatments and their usefulness in the street medicine setting.

References

1. The California Statewide Study of People Experiencing Homelessness Toward a New Understanding. 2023.
2. Su KY, Feldman BJ, Feldman CT, Saluja S, Coulourides Kogan AM, Cousineau MR. Behavioral health care delivery through street medicine programs in California. Community Ment Health J. 2024;60(2):283–91.
3. Health Conditions Among Unsheltered Adults in the U.S_.
4. Richards J, Kuhn R. Unsheltered homelessness and health: a literature review. Vol. 2, AJPM Focus. Elsevier B.V.; 2023.
5. Roncarati JS, Baggett TP, O'Connell JJ, Hwang SW, Francis Cook E, Krieger N, et al. Mortality among unsheltered homeless adults in Boston, Massachusetts, 2000–2009. In: JAMA Internal Medicine. American Medical Association; 2018. p. 1231–1240.
6. Wen CK, Hudak PL, Hwang SW. Homeless People's Perceptions of Welcomeness and Unwelcomeness in Healthcare Encounters. J Gen Intern Med [Internet]. 2007 [cited 2025 May 8];22(7):1011. Available from: https://pmc.ncbi.nlm.nih.gov/articles/PMC2219712/
7. Gilmer C, Buccieri K. Homeless Patients Associate Clinician Bias With Suboptimal Care for Mental Illness, Addictions, and Chronic Pain. J Prim Care Community Health [Internet]. 2020 [cited 2025 May 8];11:2150132720910289. Available from: https://pmc.ncbi.nlm.nih.gov/articles/PMC7059226/
8. Hoffman L, Coffey B. Dignity and indignation: how people experiencing homelessness view services and providers. Soc Sci J [Internet] 2008 [cited 2025 May 8];45(2):207–222. Available from: https://www.tandfonline.com/doi/pdf/10.1016/j.soscij.2008.03.001
9. Street Medicine for Unsheltered Individuals: Serving People Where They Are. 2021.
10. Our Vision & Mission [Internet]. [cited 2025 May 8]. Available from: https://www.streetmedicine.org/our-vision-mission
11. Collins SE, Clifasefi SL, Nelson LA, Stanton J, Goldstein SC, Taylor EM, et al. Randomized controlled trial of harm reduction treatment for alcohol (HaRT-A) for people experiencing homelessness and alcohol use disorder. International J Drug Policy [Internet]. 2019 [cited 2025 May 8];67:24–33. Available from: https://pubmed.ncbi.nlm.nih.gov/30851620/
12. Collins SE, Jones CB, Hoffmann G, Nelson LA, Hawes SM, Grazioli VS, et al. In their own words: Content analysis of pathways to recovery among individuals with the lived experience of homelessness and alcohol use disorders. International Journal of Drug Policy [Internet]. 2016 [cited 2025 May 8];27:89–96. Available from: https://www.sciencedirect.com/science/article/abs/pii/S0955395915002388?via%3Dihub
13. O'Shaughnessy BR, Mayock P, Kakar A. The recovery experiences of homeless service users with substance use disorder: A systematic review and qualitative meta-synthesis. Int J Drug Policy [Internet]. 2024 [cited 2025 May 8];130:104528. Available from: https://www.sciencedirect.com/science/article/pii/S0955395924002135
14. What is Harm Reduction? – Harm Reduction International [Internet]. [cited 2025 May 6]. Available from: https://hri.global/what-is-harm-reduction/
15. Drug Decriminalization in Portugal: Lessons for Creating Fair and Successful Drug Policies | Cato Institute [Internet]. [cited 2025 May 6]. Available from: https://www.cato.org/white-paper/drug-decriminalization-portugal-lessons-creating-fair-successful-drug-policies

16. Killias M, Aebi MF. The impact of heroin prescription on heroin markets in Switzerland. Crime Prevent Stud. 2000;11:83–99.
17. Platt L, Minozzi S, Reed J, Vickerman P, Hagan H, French C, et al. Needle syringe programmes and opioid substitution therapy for preventing hepatitis C transmission in people who inject drugs. Cochrane Database Syst Rev [Internet] 2017 [cited 2025 May 6];9(9). Available from: https://pubmed.ncbi.nlm.nih.gov/28922449/
18. Mattick RP, Breen C, Kimber J, Davoli M. Methadone maintenance therapy versus no opioid replacement therapy for opioid dependence. Cochrane Database of Systematic Reviews [Internet] 2009 [cited 2025 May 6];(3). Available from: https://www.cochranelibrary.com/cdsr/doi/10.1002/14651858.CD002209.pub2/full
19. Marshall BD, Milloy MJ, Wood E, Montaner JS, Kerr T. Reduction in overdose mortality after the opening of North America's first medically supervised safer injecting facility: a retrospective population-based study. Lancet [Internet] 2011 [cited 2025 May 6];377(9775):1429–1437. Available from: https://pubmed.ncbi.nlm.nih.gov/21497898/
20. Walley AY, Xuan Z, Hackman HH, Quinn E, Doe-Simkins M, Sorensen-Alawad A, et al. Opioid overdose rates and implementation of overdose education and nasal naloxone distribution in Massachusetts: interrupted time series analysis. BMJ [Internet]. 2013 [cited 2025 May 6];346(7894). Available from: https://www.bmj.com/content/346/bmj.f174
21. Ledlie S, Garg R, Cheng C, Kolla G, Antoniou T, Bouck Z, et al. Prescribed safer opioid supply: a scoping review of the evidence. Int J Drug Policy. 2024;125:104339.
22. Slaunwhite A, Min JE, Palis H, Urbanoski K, Pauly B, Barker B, et al. Effect of risk mitigation guidance for opioid and stimulant dispensations on mortality and acute care visits during dual public health emergencies: retrospective cohort study. BMJ [Internet] 2024 [cited 2025 May 4];384. Available from: https://www.bmj.com/CONTENT/384/BMJ-2023-076336

6 Medication Treatment of Substance Use Disorders

6.1 Introduction

Whereas the last chapter focused on guiding principles of substance use disorder care, this chapter examines drugs and alcohol that street medicine patients commonly use, methods to harm reduction associated with using each substance, treatment for ill effects of intoxication and withdrawal, and treatments, where available, to help patients reduce or quit using if it is their goal.

Polysubstance use is the norm in the street medicine setting and very few street medicine patients who use drugs only use one or one at a time. Most patients do have one or a few preferred substances they regularly use, however, and use others more intermittently. Cannabis, tobacco, and alcohol use are standard among patients and not uncommon among street medicine clinicians. Though the health issues facing people sleeping rough are often incredibly clinically complex, street medicine typically affords clinicians the time, flexibility, and team support to they need to provide high-quality patient care and enjoy the work.

Table 6.1 summarizes substances that street medicine patients may use, though it is not an exhaustive list. There are many more street names for drugs than are listed in Table 6.1; if your patient mentions a drug or street name with which you are unfamiliar, just ask them what it is. Street medicine patients are excellent educators related to drugs and alcohol—likely far better than you or I—and typically do not mind sharing their knowledge.

S. Hatcher et al., *Street Mental Health Handbook*,
https://doi.org/10.1007/978-3-032-00663-9_6

Table 6.1 Substances used on the streets

Drug name	Examples & other names	Methods of use	Desired effect
Alcohol	Beer, wine, liquor, malt liquor	Oral	Relaxation, reduced anxiety, sedation
Benzodiazepines	Xanax, Klonopin	Oral	Relaxation, reduced anxiety, sedation
Cannabis / synthetic cannabinoids	Marijuana/ K2, spice	Smoked	Relaxation, reduced anxiety, appetite stimulant
Cocaine	Crack	Snorted, smoked (crack), injected	Euphoria, increased energy, increased alertness and focus
Methamphetamine	Meth, crystal meth	Smoked (crystal meth), injected, oral	Euphoria, increased energy, increased alertness and focus, increased sex drive
Opioids	Heroin, fentanyl	Snorted, smoked, injected, oral	Relaxation, sedation, pain relief
Psychedelics	MDMA (ecstasy), psylocibin, LSD, PCP, peyote,	Smoked, snorted, injected	Altered sense of reality & connectedness, hallucinations
Synthetic Cathinones	Bath salts	Snorted, injected	Euphoria, increased alertness and energy
Tranquilizers	Xylazine, medetomidine, ketamine	Oral, injected	Reduced anxiety, calm
Tobacco	Cigarettes, cigars, loose tobacco	Smoked, chewed	Calm, more alert

6.2 Interviews with Street Medicine Clinicians

For assistance with this chapter and the previous chapter, I informally interviewed street medicine clinicians working in the United States (U.S.) who I know through work with the Street Medicine Institute or who were recommended to me as experts in street-based addiction medicine. My coauthors shared information about common interventions and practices in Canada and their experiences working in street medicine in Ottawa. There are very few publications related to treating and preventing harm from problematic substance use in the street medicine setting or that focus primarily on interventions for people sleeping rough. These informal interviews with street medicine clinicians were not intended as scientific research and do not meet criteria for it. Rather, during the interviews, I attempted to gather information on what and how street medicine clinicians are doing, despite the paucity of research, to care for people sleeping rough with incredibly complex physical, mental, and substance use disorders. I present information from my interviews, my own practices, and information from research about substance use treatment in the street medicine setting as well as research on substance use and interventions in various unsheltered, sheltered, and housed populations where available. I was impressed with how much variability exists from city to city—even within neighborhoods—in commonly used drugs, contamination in the drug supply, community resource availability, policies and laws that impact people using drugs, and what capacity different street medicine teams have to implement interventions. From my perspective, the only clear gold-standard practices for problematic substance use in the street medicine setting are harm reduction, letting our patients take the lead and set the goals, and willingness to accompany people on their journeys whatever choices they make. Hopefully, you will find the information in this chapter and the next chapter useful in weighing the risks and benefits of various treatment options, considering how to tailor interventions for the streets, and determining what practices align with your team's values and risk tolerance in the unique setting where you work.

6.3 Clinician Philosophies on Diversion, Discharge, Drug Screens, and Therapy

Clinicians interviewed for this chapter and the next chapter have varying philosophies about requirements for prescribing controlled medications for substance use disorders. All take a very low-threshold harm-reduction compassionate approach. Many street medicine clinicians feel indifferent about diversion of buprenorphine from a public health standpoint, noting that when prescriptions are sold, the buyer is almost always another person with opioid use disorder. All recognized, however, that diversion is harmful for the patient they are treating and expressed desire for the patient not to divert. The single discharge from opioid use disorder (OUD) care mentioned occurred when the team discovered a patient was in treatment at a methadone clinic, preferred methadone, and was selling his buprenorphine prescriptions for survival money. The team continued care, however, for the patient's other health concerns.

Urine drug screens were the most controversial—some clinicians hate them and never test, some find them annoying and test irregularly, others find them valuable and test whenever they follow up with the patient for OUD. No one required a UDS unless a private restroom was available, typically in a clinical setting. Clinicians who value them reported the test being a useful discussion tool and use them as a "vital sign" of how well recovery is going. One clinician expressed the view that lying to oneself and others is a symptom of substance use disorders and believes that urine drug screens promote honest conversations that benefit both the patient and the clinician. None of the street medicine clinicians interviewed had discontinued care for a patient due to a positive urine drug screen. Some clinicians said that they had stopped prescribing buprenorphine after five or more weekly prescriptions if the patient's UDS was never positive for buprenorphine, but attempted to continue caring for the patient in every other possible way. These clinicians were almost always happy to retry induction if the patient expressed readiness. Clinicians who regularly collect a UDS occasionally send the urine to test for buprenorphine metabolites. Most clinicians rarely use saliva swabs.

Most clinicians interviewed believe that best substance use disorder care involves therapy or other psychosocial interventions, but only one made it a requirement of treatment and offered interventions in a convenient location for most patients. Most clinicians have few options to refer patient for therapy interventions, such as trauma therapy, that they felt was important to recovery. Some clinicians expressed wanting to hire someone to provide therapy for their street medicine patients and funding restrictions were the primary reason for not hiring someone. Street psychiatry teams are more likely to offer therapy than primary care street medicine teams, even though every primary care clinician interviewed treats mental health conditions ranging from depression to psychosis on the street.

While there are many well-studied treatments for various substance use disorders (SUD), there is a paucity of evidence for treatments in the street medicine setting or treatments focused solely on people living unsheltered. This chapter summarizes the desired and ill effects of commonly used substances among street medicine patients, methods to reduce the harmful impacts of these substances, treatment options, and common practices among street medicine teams within the United States and Canada. This chapter does not focus on how to make a substance use disorder diagnosis, as the diagnosis itself is less important than understanding what a person is using, how to reduce harm from using, and how to help patients cut back or quit if they are interested. The text does use the term "substance use disorder" or specific disorders, as the majority of street medicine clinicians do not perform formal assessments to determine if their patients meet DSM criteria for the SUD.

6.4 Psychosocial Interventions and Therapy

There are multiple kinds of interventions and therapies that are useful in the treatment of substance use disorders, including Cognitive Behavioral Therapy (CBT), Motivational Enhancement Therapy (also called Motivational Interviewing), Acceptance- and mindfulness-based interventions, and Contingency Management. While not an intervention specific to SUD, trauma therapy is vital for a large portion of people living unsheltered, as many are affected by the sequelae of trauma. For people with post-traumatic stress disorder (PTSD) and other trauma-stressor disorders, trauma therapy can be substantially more impactful for reducing alcohol use—even when substance use is not addressed—than interventions focused on substance use. See Chap. 11 for details of psychosocial interventions.

6.5 Alcohol

Alcohol use disorder is common among people who are homeless, affecting 53–73%, both before and after becoming homeless [1]. People who are homeless and drink alcohol daily are two times more likely to live unsheltered, placing them at higher risk of death [2]. Roncarati and colleagues found that people living unsheltered in Boston were 110 times more likely to die from alcohol use disorder than the general

Massachusetts population, accounting for 22% of deaths in the unsheltered cohort. Further, the unsheltered cohort was 32 and 4.5 times more likely to die from chronic liver disease than the general and sheltered populations respectively [3]. These deaths were most likely caused by chronic alcohol use and untreated Hepatitis C.

In a 2023 qualitative study in Montreal, people sleeping rough report drinking alcohol to cope with conditions of the street, such as to warm up and sleep and to cope with emotional distress. Most participants reported wanting to escape the reality of been seen as "trash" as well as use it as "medicine to forget the past," including childhood abuse, intimate partner violence, loss of loved ones, and being victimized on the streets. Further, alcohol is seen as part of the culture of the streets, a way to make friends, and be a part of a community [4].

6.5.1 Reducing Harm from Alcohol Use

In order to reduce harm from alcohol use, start with learning how much and what kind of alcohol your patient drinks. Typically, drinking regular beer with less than seven percent alcohol content or "alcohol by volume" (ABV) is lower risk and consuming alcohol in the form of mouthwash or hand sanitizer is higher risk. Figure 6.1 shows the spectrum of risk based on alcohol type [5].

Harm reduction with alcohol use typically includes encouragement not to consume non-beverage alcohol, such as hand sanitizer and mouthwash. Consuming enough of these products to become drunk typically includes consuming toxic levels of other chemicals, which is why they are particularly harmful. Other harm reduction methods include assistance in drinking smaller cans of beer or beer with a lower alcohol content, encouragement to drink water and eat while drinking alcohol, and avoid drinking and using other substances at the same time [6]. When thinking about the harms of an individual's alcohol use, get creative to mitigate the harms. If a patient drinks sufficient amounts of beer to cause seizures from hyponatremia, encouraging them to switch to liquor may reduce harm. Remind street

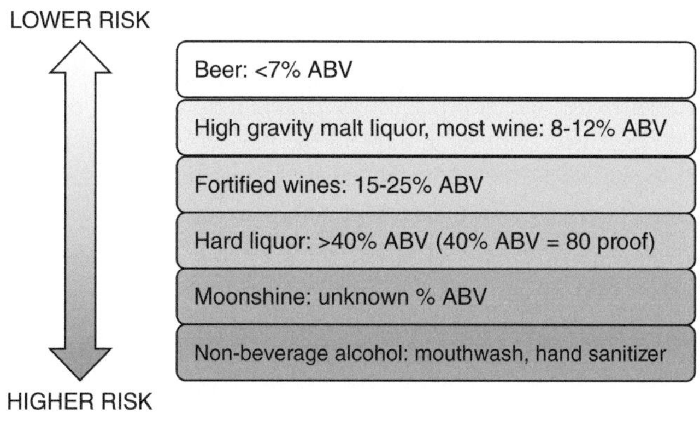

Fig. 6.1 Risk associated with alcohol type

medicine patients get in their sleeping bags before drinking on cold or rainy nights. Alcohol can make them feel warmer than they are and getting in their sleeping bags first prevents hypothermia and death.

All patients with problematic alcohol use should be prescribed vitamins to reduce the harm of alcohol use, including thiamine (B1), folate, and B12. A daily multivitamin is also ideal. Thiamine 100 mg daily is particularly important to prevent neurological problems such as Wernicke-Korsakoff syndrome. Folate and B12 deficiencies are common among people with problematic alcohol use, due to impaired absorption. If your patient is willing, prescribe folate 1 mg daily and B12 100 mg daily. Patients found to have macrocytic anemia on complete blood count may need higher doses or an injection for B-12 deficiency.

Managed alcohol programs (MAPs) are gaining in popularity as an option for reducing alcohol-related harms among unhoused people with severe alcohol use disorder, particularly among people for whom abstinence is not a goal. Managed alcohol programs provide individuals with regular doses of alcohol in a supportive living environment. Shannon Bernardin-Smith, a street medicine nurse practitioner, and colleagues published a scoping review of managed alcohol programs in 2022. Compared to people in the shelter-based treatment-as-usual control groups, participants in MAPs were less likely to report seizures, acute intoxication, trauma, or assault due to alcohol use and reported significantly less overall alcohol consumption. Non-beverage alcohol use was significantly reduced among MAP participants. Unsurprisingly, MAPs that had more stringent rules related to outside alcohol consumption demonstrated significantly fewer alcohol-related harms among participants compared to controls. MAPs with no or less stringent rules did not have statistically significant reductions in harms. MAP participants reported higher quality of life on four domains—physical, psychological, relationships, and environments—though only environment was significantly higher [7].

6.5.2 Symptoms of Alcohol Intoxication

Though most people are familiar with symptoms of alcohol intoxication, they include confusion, slurred words or being unable to speak, problems with coordination such as difficulty standing/walking and picking things up, vomiting, loss of control of bowel or bladder, falling asleep, blackouts, and loss of consciousness. Blackouts are described as missing gaps in the person's memory and are different from falling asleep and loss of consciousness. Typically, the person is awake and functioning to some degree, but has no memory of it later. Blackouts tend to occur more often when the blood alcohol level rises quickly [8].

6.5.3 Evaluation and Management of Alcohol Withdrawal

Alcohol withdrawal symptoms can occur at any blood alcohol level, depending on the average amount of alcohol a person generally consumes. Alcohol withdrawal occurs when someone who is physiologically dependent either chooses to drink much less or is unable to drink their normal amount. Symptoms include tremors, sweating, anxiety, nausea, vomiting, insomnia, tachycardia, hypertension, psychomotor agitation, and hyperventilation and can progress to seizures, hallucinations, and delirium tremens [9]. Psychological withdrawal includes cravings and using dreams.

Dr. Andie Silva, a double board-certified physician in Addiction Medicine and Family Medicine and clinical professor at University of California Davis, is the founder and medical director of Valley Streetz, a street medicine and harm reduction organization in Modesto, CA. She recommends using the Prediction of Alcohol Withdrawal Severity Scale (PAWSS) when assessing likelihood that a person sleeping outside will develop complicated alcohol withdrawal syndrome, such as seizures and DTs. Though the PAWSS was developed to predict complicated withdrawal among medically ill hospitalized patients, it can make an excellent history-taking tool when considering the level of care a street medicine patient may need if they want to stop drinking or are forced to stop drinking due to hospitalization or incarceration. With a positive score of four or more, PAWSS has 93.1% sensitivity and 99.5% specificity in predicting complicated withdrawal. Scores of less than four have a negative predictive value of 99.5%, indicating uncomplicated withdrawal in which the person will likely only need supportive medical intervention [10].

Patients who have a PAWSS score less than four and who have mild to moderate alcohol use disorder, street-based unsupervised management may be possible. Use your clinical judgment to determine if your patient has sufficient cognitive capacity to follow the protocol or if they have a friend who is able to help out. Depending on your patient, your relationship with them, your level of comfort, and possibly the patient or a friend's ability to read, you may consider prescribing street-based withdrawal medications either only when you find the person in withdrawal, in advance of a planned withdrawal, or for a future "just-in-case" scenario in which the person is unable to obtain alcohol and goes into withdrawal. Street medicine patients who live in secluded or rural areas where there is limited access to emergency medicine services (EMS) or "ambulance deserts" may benefit from access to protocol medications for unplanned withdrawal. See Table 6.2 for a benzodiazepine-sparing protocol that Dr. Andie Silva developed. Use the protocol only for patients with mild to moderate alcohol use disorder with PAWSS score less than four.

For patients in withdrawal who are not interested in medication treatment, are not trying to stop drinking, or who do not want go to the emergency room, some street medicine clinicians purchase and provide them with alcohol to avoid complications of alcohol withdrawal. All patients with a PAWSS score of four or greater who want to stop drinking, should be directed to the hospital for management of withdrawal. With advance planning, street medicine teams may be able to coordinate with friendly inpatient addiction medicine consult services or friendly inpatient physicians to plan for inpatient alcohol withdrawal management for street medicine patients wishing to stop drinking. Street medicine patients who need or want psychiatric admission may need to undergo inpatient medical detox first if they have a history of complicated withdrawal.

Table 6.2 Outpatient unsupervised withdrawal protocol

Prescribe all of the following medications if there are no contraindications		
Medication	Dose	Frequency
Gabapentin (Neurontin)	600–800 mg	TID × 5 days
Valproic acid (Depakote)	500 mg	BID × 2 weeks
Clonidine (Catapres)	0.1 mg	QID PRN anxiety
Odansetron (Zofran)	4 mg	Q4–6 hours PRN nausea/vomiting

Table 6.3 Medication treatment for alcohol use disorder

Medication	Dosing	Common side effects	Other
Acamprosate (Campral)	666 mg po TID	Diarrhea	Start 3–5 days after last drink, but abstinence is not required
Disulfiram (Antabuse)	500 mg po Qam × 2 weeks, then may lower to 250 mg or 125 mg daily	Strange aftertaste, fatigue, headache, sexual dysfunction	Start at least 12–24 hours after last drink when completely sober. Abstinence is required
Naltrexone oral (Revia)	25 mg po Qam × 3 days, then 50 mg po Qam	Abdominal pain, anxiety, insomnia, nausea, vomiting, fatigue	Abstinence is not required
Naltrexone extended-release injection (Vivitrol)	380 mg IM Q4 weeks (gluteal only)	Abdominal pain, anxiety, insomnia, nausea, vomiting, fatigue, pain/swelling at injection site	Test safety with at least one oral naltrexone dose first. Abstinence is not required.
Topiramate (Topamax)	Start 25 mg po BID and increase by 25 mg BID once weekly to 75 or 100 mg BID. Increase to 150 mg po BID after a week of 100 mg BID. Maintenance dose is 75 to 150 mg po BID.	Significant cognitive impairment, nausea, sedation, muscle tremors, dizziness, reduced appetite or weight loss	Abstinence is not required

6.5.4 Medication Treatment for Alcohol Use Disorder

Patients who are interested in medication treatment to stop drinking or cut down have a few options: acamprosate (Campral), oral naltrexone (Revia), extended-release injectable naltrexone (Vivitrol), topiramate (Topamax), and disulfiram (Antabuse). Generally, acamprosate and naltrexone are considered first line and disulfiram is a second-line treatment. As with all medication treatment in the street medicine setting, carefully weigh the risks and benefits of medication as well as the risks of remaining on the street due to lack of treatment. Make sure the medication choice matches your patient's goals. Prescribing information for each of these medications is listed in Table 6.3.

6.5.4.1 Naltrexone (Revia, Vivitrol)

Most street medicine clinicians prefer injectable naltrexone to other treatments for patients who do not use opioids because of its dosing every four weeks and relatively few side effects compared with other medications. Injectable naltrexone needs to be refrigerated, but can be left out of the refrigerator for a maximum of seven days prior to administration. Oral naltrexone is used as an alternative for patients who do not want to receive injections, though most clinicians report better outcomes for street medicine patients taking the injection. Naltrexone works by reducing the pleasurable effects of alcohol. Patients whose goals do not include cessation of alcohol use will likely prefer naltrexone, as they can still drink while taking naltrexone and sobriety is not required to start naltrexone. Better outcomes may be more likely, however, if naltrexone is started during abstinence [11]. Studies of naltrexone in the general population indicate it has moderate-strength evidence for reducing return to drinking and return to heavy drinking as well as lowering percentage of drinking days and heaving drinking days compared to placebo [12]. Naltrexone is contraindicated for people using opioids and for liver function tests five times the normal limit.

6.5.4.2 Acamprosate (Campral)

Acamprosate works by reducing the desire to drink and is associated with improvement in alcohol consumption outcomes similar to naltrexone [12]. It has a significantly larger effect size than naltrexone for maintenance of abstinence, but is less effective for cravings and reduction of heavy drinking compared to naltrexone [13]. Acamprosate, similar to naltrexone, does not require abstinence to start, though better outcomes occur when started after three to five days of not consuming alcohol. It can be continued if patients return to drinking. Acamprosate has a high pill burden; it is dosed as two 333 mg pills three times daily, limiting its usefulness in the street medicine setting. Acamprosate is contraindicated for renal insufficiency, but is an alternative for people with liver disease [13].

6.5.4.3 Topiramate (Topamax)

Topiramate works by reducing cravings for alcohol and has moderate strength of evidence of statistically significant improvement in reducing the percentage of drinking days and heavy drinking days, as well as the number of drinks per day compared with placebo [12]. Topiramate is associated with cognitive dysfunction limiting its use on the street given the heavy burden of cognitive dysfunction among people sleeping rough. While some clinicians use it for treatment of bipolar disorder, it is typically less effective than other treatments mentioned in Chap. 4 of this handbook. Topiramate reduces the effectiveness of hormonal contraceptives, including oral and patch contraceptives, the emergency contraceptive levonorgestrel (plan B), vaginal rings, injections, and implants.

6.5.4.4 Disulfiram (Antabuse)

Many street medicine clinicians are hesitant to prescribe disulfiram due to concern for its effects if a patient consumes alcohol intentionally while taking disulfiram.

Patients can accidentally consume or come into contact with small amounts of alcohol in toothpaste, deodorant, some over-the-counter cold medications, sauces containing vinegar, some transdermal patches, and alcohol skin wipes. With touching these products, patients taking disulfiram may develop headache, nausea, and local redness or itching of the skin. Even breathing certain chemicals, such as paint thinner, can induce a reaction. With consumption of alcohol, the disulfiram reaction includes blurred vision, chest pain, confusion, dizziness and fainting, tachycardia, flushing or redness of the face, increased sweating, nausea, vomiting, throbbing headache, difficulty breathing, and weakness. The reactions will last as long as alcohol is in the body, anywhere from 30 minutes to several hours and the severity of the reaction typically depends on the amount of alcohol consumed. A severe reaction including unconsciousness, seizures, myocardial infarction, and death may occur with intentional consumption of large amounts of alcohol [14]. These symptoms are exactly the purpose of taking disulfiram; when patients know that drinking on disulfiram is incredibly uncomfortable and possibly deadly, they usually do not drink. Even when patients stop taking disulfiram, they may experience a disulfiram reaction when exposed to alcohol up to two weeks later. Instruct patients to start disulfiram only after abstaining from alcohol for at least 12 hours. Disulfiram is typically started at 500 mg once daily for two weeks. The maintenance dose can be decreased to 250 mg or 125 mg daily or continued at 500 mg. Do not exceed 500 mg daily.

6.6 Benzodiazepines

Benzodiazepines (benzos) largely have the same effects as alcohol, though problematic alcohol use among people living unsheltered is far more common. Detection of benzos in U.S. drug samples increased significantly starting in 2018 and may have reached a plateau in 2022. In many places, benzodiazepines are sold online and on the streets as counterfeit Xanax pills and have little in common with prescription benzos. As of 2024, most contain designer benzodiazepines (DBZ) such as bromazolam, rilmazafone, and clonazolam [15]. "Benzo-dope," pills (opioids adulterated with benzodiazepines) were first identified in Canada in 2020 and have become increasingly common in the United States. DBZs are cheap, widely available, and enhance the effects of fentanyl, which is why suppliers cut DBZs into the fentanyl supply. In the U.S. and Canada, overdose deaths with benzos and DBZs usually involve opioids. Standard urine drug screens often do not detect DBZs.

6.6.1 Reducing Harm from Benzodiazepine Use

Harm reduction options include test strips, safe injection supplies for benzos being injected, and supervised consumption facilities that monitor vital signs and help people use more slowly. Safer supply for benzos is offered in some places in Canada [16]. There are benzodiazepine test strips that can detect some DBZs and are being used in supervised consumption sites in Canada. Given the ever-evolving nature of synthetic designer benzos, test strips technology must continue to evolve as well.

6.6.2 Benzodiazepine Intoxication and Withdrawal

The desired effects of benzodiazepines include feeling calm, relaxed, and drowsy. DBZs have similar anti-anxiety properties, but can be twice as potent or more. Depending on the specific DBZ, the most prominent feature may be anxiolysis, euphoria, amnesia, or hypnotic. Intoxication with all benzodiazepines looks similar to alcohol intoxication with slurred speech, ataxia, altered mental status, and sedation. Other negative effects include problems with memory, confusion, headaches, fainting, nausea, vomiting, diarrhea, and tremors. Overdose of benzos typically causes altered mental status, sedation, nystagmus, decreased deep tendon reflexes, hypotension, hypotonia, and respiratory depression, but may also cause respiratory failure, seizures, coma, and death. Withdrawal symptoms are similar to alcohol including anxiety, tremor, delirium, agitation, and psychosis [17]. The clinical picture of DBZs includes heavy hypnosis and sedation, long-lasting amnesia, rapid tolerance, and longer-lasting withdrawal. Flumazenil is a weak partial benzodiazepine agonist and is approved for overdose, but is contraindicated in unknown or mixed overdoses. Flumazenil can also be used to manage benzodiazepine withdrawal, as can longer-acting benzodiazepines [15].

6.6.3 Medication Treatment for Benzodiazepine Use Disorder

Treatment benzodiazepine use disorder is underexplored. Options typically include management of withdrawal with a plan for abstinence or prescribed benzodiazepine maintenance therapy. Psychotherapies and medication treatment for cooccurring anxiety disorders offer some successes. A small 2022 study evaluated flumazenil infusions of four milligrams over 24 hours for eight days given during withdrawal and followed patients at one, two, and three months. Abstinence rates were high, with 61.5% at three months. A 2014 study suggested that low-dose flumazenil could be used for maintenance treatment of benzodiazepines either as a depot injection or implant, though there are none of these options available on the market and it is unclear if there will be [18]. The usefulness of flumazenil treatment is likely low for street medicine patients, however, given that most people using benzodiazepines are using them concomitantly with opioids and other drugs. Treatments for alcohol use disorder have not been well explored for benzodiazepine use disorder, but they do not appear to reduce cravings for benzodiazepines.

6.7 Cannabis and Synthetic Cannabinoids (K2, Spice)

Roughly half of people who are homeless use cannabis [19]. Young unsheltered individuals are over two times more likely to use synthetic cannabinoids than their sheltered counterparts [20]. Offering relief from anxiety and pain, relaxation, elevated mood, and a heightened sense of well-being, it is easy to understand why unsheltered people would use cannabis. As the majority of street medicine patients cannot afford medical-grade cannabis, they commonly consume contaminated cannabis. A 2025 Canadian analysis found that most illegal product samples contained levels of heavy metals, mycotoxins, pesticides, bacteria species above the United States Pharmacopeia tolerance limit set for inhalation [21, 22]. No medication treatment exists for cannabis/ synthetic cannabinoid use disorder.

6.7.1 Reducing Harm from Cannabis Use

Incarceration due to cannabis possession could arguably cause the highest health consequences among unsheltered individuals in the United States. Street medicine clinicians may choose to authorize medical marijuana cards for patients as a harm reduction measure and even among patients with psychotic disorders. Additionally, in 2019 the Centers for Disease Control and Prevention documented numerous hospitalizations and 68 deaths related lung injury after vaping cannabis containing the chemical vitamin E acetate [23]. Encouraging street medicine patients to avoid vaping cannabis products also reduces harm.

6.7.2 Cannabis Intoxication and Withdrawal

Short-term undesired effects include amotivation, anxiety, paranoia, irritability, restlessness, distrust, and hallucinations. Long-term cannabis can lead to respiratory problems; increased risk for arrhythmias, myocardial infarction, and stroke; cannabinoid hyperemesis syndrome; and increased risk of head, neck, and throat cancer. Cannabis use can also cause earlier onset and worsened psychosis among people with genetic risk for psychotic disorders [24]. Withdrawal symptoms include irritability, aggression, anxiety, restlessness, decreased appetite, insomnia, strange dreams, nausea, vomiting, and abdominal pain. Roughly half of regular users experience withdrawal [25].

6.7.3 Synthetic Cannabinoid Intoxication and Withdrawal

Synthetic cannabinoids, more commonly referred to as K2 or spice, contain high levels of THC and place people sleeping outside at much higher risk of death compared to cannabis. Studies of K2 use in the UK among people who are homeless report that the majority are using K2 to escape the reality of homelessness or to self-medicate [26]. Synthetic cannabinoids, like cannabis are typically smoked and have similar desired and undesired effects as cannabis intoxication, only stronger. Milder toxicity symptoms include agitation, drowsiness, nausea, vomiting, tachycardia, hypertension, psychosis, muscle twitches, respiratory depression, and muscle twitching. People with moderate to severe toxidrome develop more dangerous symptoms of seizures, delirium, unconsciousness, respiratory depression requiring ventilator support, acute cardiac toxicity, acute renal failure, and acute hepatic injury that can result in death [27]. Withdrawal symptoms are similar to cannabis, but more severe.

6.8 Cocaine

Fatal overdoses involving cocaine tripled from 2012 to 2021, increasing an average 21% per year, in part due to the increasing use of cocaine and other stimulants among people who use opioids and the rise of fentanyl contaminants in the cocaine and crack supply. While the rates of cocaine use have been almost flat, cocaine use disorder is becoming more common. In 2021, 23% of all overdose deaths involved cocaine [28].

Cocaine is consumed by snorting, injecting, and smoking (crack). Its desired effects include euphoria, increased energy, increased socialization, and alertness. Ill effects include irritability, restlessness, anxiety, paranoia, hallucinations, headaches, insomnia, formication, delusional parasitosis, movement disorders, and both acute and long-term cardiovascular and neurologic effects. The movement disorders—cocaine-induced hyperkinesis—include tics, dystonia, essential tremor, myoclonus, and choreathetosis similar to bath salts. Long-term cocaine and crack users may develop tardive dyskinesia.

6.8.1 Reducing Harm from Cocaine/Crack Use

Harm reduction for snorting, injecting, and smoking cocaine largely relies on safe use supplies. Safe snorting supplies include a faux razor made of hard plastic, a personal Pyrex straw or straight stem to prevent spread of infectious pathogens, and sterile water for rinsing the nose. Switching nostrils regularly helps reduce damage and irritation to the nostril. Safe smoking supplies include a glass or metal stem to use as a pipe, a personal plastic mouthpiece, and chore (made from copper kitchen scrubbers). The personal plastic mouthpiece protects users from burns and open sores. Safe shooting (injecting) supplies include sterile cookers, water, cotton, and needles/syringes in addition to vitamin C (ascorbic acid to dissolve the cocaine) tourniquet. Users should clean their hands and supplies with alcohol wipes before each use to prevent bacterial contamination. Personal supplies help users avoid sharing, which makes them more vulnerable to HIV and hepatitis C infection. Techniques for shooting straight, or hitting the vein, are important. Users should avoid injecting veins in their genitals.

6.8.2 Cocaine Toxicity

Acute toxicity with cocaine has three phases. In fatal cases, onset and progression are accelerated and death can occur in as few as two or three minutes or as many as 30 minutes. See Table 6.4 for symptoms during each phase [29]. Treatment begins with benzodiazepines for central nervous system (CNS) effects and medications to control cardiovascular effects. Fluid resuscitation for rhabdomyolysis and submersion in an ice bath for hyperthermia follow if patients outlive the CNS and cardiovascular effects of acute toxicity.

Table 6.4 Phases of acute cocaine toxicity

Phase 1	CNS: mydriasis, headache, bruxism, nausea, vomiting, vertigo, twitching of facial and finger muscles, tics, hallucinations
	Circulatory: possible elevations in blood pressure and pulse, pallor
	Respiratory: increased rate and depth
	Temperature: mildly elevated
	Behavioral: euphoria, elation, garrulous talk, agitation, apprehension, excitation, restlessness, verbalization of impending doom, and emotional lability
Phase 2	CNS: malignant encephalopathy, seizures, decreased responsiveness to all stimuli, hyperreflexia, incontinence
	Circulatory: hypertension, tachycardia, possible ventricular dysrhythmias (resulting in weak, rapid, irregular pulse and hypotension), peripheral cyanosis
	Respiratory: tachypnea, dyspnea, gasping, and irregular breathing
	Temperature: severe hyperthermia
Phase 3	CNS: Coma, areflexia, pupils fixed and dilated, flaccid paralysis, and loss of vital support functions
	Circulatory: cardiovascular collapse; ventricular fibrillation or asystole
	Respiratory: respiratory failure, gross pulmonary edema, cyanosis, agonal respirations, and paralysis of respiration
	Temperature: severe hyperthermia

6.8.3 Cocaine Withdrawal

Stopping cocaine use or at the end of a binge, users experience an immediate crash characterized by intense cravings for more cocaine. Unlike withdrawal from heroin or alcohol, cocaine withdrawal typically lacks visible physical symptoms such as vomiting or tremors. Common symptoms of cocaine withdrawal include agitation and restlessness; low mood; fatigue; general discomfort; increased appetite; vivid, unpleasant dreams; and psychomotor retardation. Cravings and depression may persist for months after discontinuing long-term heavy use. Some individuals may experience suicidal ideation during withdrawal. Intense cravings for cocaine can occur throughout the withdrawal process. As ongoing use continues, the pleasurable effects of the drug may diminish, potentially leading to increased fear and anxiety.

6.8.4 Medication Treatment for Cocaine Use Disorder

Fortunately, with the rise in use and deaths associated with stimulants, researchers have invested more in discovering treatments for cocaine use disorder (CUD). None of the pharmacotherpies have been approved by the U.S. Food and Drug Administration (FDA) and all are used off label. All of these medications have risks in the street medicine setting that need to be weighed against untreated cocaine use disorder. Recommendations in this section come from the 2024 "ASAM/AAAP Clinical Practice Guideline on the Management of Stimulant Use Disorder," which is definitely worth a read [28]. An anti-cocaine vaccine has been in development for over 25 years, but still has not undergone any human testing.

6.8.4.1 Non-stimulant Medications for Cocaine Use Disorder

Bupropion XL (Wellbutrin XL) and topiramate (Topamax) are non-stimulant medications used for cocaine use disorder and can be prescribed while the patient is using cocaine. Bupropion XL (Wellbutrin XL) promotes cocaine abstinence is particularly recommended for cooccurring disorders including tobacco use disorder and depression, but is contraindicated for patients with any previous seizure and anorexia or bulimia. The primary concern with bupropion XL and anorexia/bulimia is electrolyte imbalance. If the patient is not restricting or purging during bupropion treatment, its risk can be weighed against the risk of continued cocaine use. Caution should also be used in prescribing bupropion for people with elevated seizure risk, which may be most patients on the streets. Topiramate (Topamax) can be helpful for reducing cocaine use and to cooccurring alcohol use disorder. It is preferred over bupropion XL for patients with a seizure history. Topiramate may be most helpful in combination with extended-release mixed amphetamine salts (Adderall XR, Mydayis) by decreasing cocaine cravings more rapidly and reducing overall cocaine use As mentioned in the section on problematic alcohol use earlier in this chapter, the cognitive impairment caused by topiramate can be substantial for people sleeping rough. See Table 6.3 in this chapter for information on prescribing topiramate. See Chap. 4, Sect. 4.6 for information regarding bupropion treatment.

6.8.4.2 Stimulant Medications for Cocaine Use Disorder

Stimulant medications used to treat CUD include modafinil (Provigil), extended-release mixed amphetamine salts (Adderall XR, Mydayis), methylphenidate, lisdexamphetamine, and dextroamphetamine. They are more helpful in treating cooccurring Attention Deficit Hyperactivity Disorder (ADHD) compared to other treatments for CUD. Each stimulant has been associated with better outcomes including reported sustained abstinence and cocaine-negative urine drug screens. Higher doses of prescription stimulants work better to treat cocaine-use disorder, including supratherapeutic doses than would be used for ADHD. If you have the ability to check an EKG, do so after starting prescribed stimulants. Longer-acting stimulants are recommended if possible. There is mixed evidence regarding modafinil treatment for cocaine use disorder, but two meta-analyses found to have a positive effect on cocaine abstinence at the end of the treatment trial. It also may be more useful for patients with higher frequency of cocaine use at the start of treatment. Modafinil interacts with and reduces the effectiveness of hormonal contraceptives. The starting dose for modafinil is 200 mg every morning. It can be increased to 300 or 400 mg, though some doses for ADHD increase above 400 mg daily. Dosing information for other stimulants listed can be found in Chap. 4, Sect. 4.8.1.2.

6.9 Methamphetamine

Methamphetamine (meth) use has become a major health hazard among people sleeping rough in North America, leaving some street medicine teams overwhelmed and dejected. Unlike opioids, there is no partial agonist medication that can be combined with medications like naloxone (Narcan) to reduce risk of misuse. Also, there is no naloxone option for methamphetamine overdose.

6.9.1 Reducing Harm from Methamphetamine Use

Harm reduction for methamphetamine use, similar to cocaine use, involves safe use supplies. The only difference in supplies for meth is that the Pyrex pipe typically has a rounded bottom for holding crystal meth, rather than a straight pipe for crack.

6.9.2 Methamphetamine Toxicity

Methamphetamine can be snorted, smoked (crystal meth), injected, and swallowed (counterfeit pressed pills). Desired effects include euphoria, increased alertness and energy, decreased appetite, confidence, increased sex drive. Adverse effects include headaches, insomnia, irritability, formication and resulting skin sores, paranoia, hallucinations, anxiety, weight loss, tooth decay and loss, hypertension, and tachycardia. Other serious effects include heart disease and failure, aortic dissection and aneurysm, pulmonary edema and pulmonary hypertension, movement disorders, prolonged psychosis, delusional parasitosis, stroke, ischemic colitis, and renal failure. The movement disorders are the same as those with cocaine use described in Sect. 6.7 of this chapter. Injecting methamphetamine can result in soft tissue infections, abscesses, and endocarditis. Methamphetamine toxicity results in the same sympathomimetic toxidrome as other stimulants including bath salts and cocaine. See Table 6.4 in Sect. 6.7.1 of this chapter for details of the toxidrome.

6.9.3 Methamphetamine Withdrawal

Abrupt withdrawal from chronic use of methamphetamines can be protracted. In the first 12 to 24 hours patients experience somnolence and dysphoric, irritable mood. The post-acute withdrawal phase can last weeks to months and may include fatigue, vivid unpleasant dreams, insomnia or hypersomnia, increased appetite, and psychomotor agitation or retardation. During this time, some people experience suicidal ideation. It may take six months to one year to fully recover from cognitive deficits and affective symptoms of withdrawal. A systematic review and meta-analysis evaluated treatments for methamphetamine withdrawal including mirtazapine (Remeron), modafinil (Provigil), varenicline (Chantix), and amantadine (Symmetrel, Gocovri); none were effective [30]. Symptomatic withdrawal treatment includes over-the-counter (OTC) pain medications for muscle aches, OTC or prescription medications for insomnia, antipsychotics, and antidepressants as needed.

6.9.4 Medication Treatment for Methamphetamine Use Disorder

Similar to treatments for cocaine use disorder, this section summarizes recommendations from the 2024 "ASAM/AAAP Clinical Practice Guideline on the Management of Stimulant Use Disorder." [28]. Both stimulants and non-stimulants have demonstrated some effectiveness with problematic methamphetamine use and none are without risks in the street medicine setting.

6.9.4.1 Non-stimulant Medications for Methamphetamine Use Disorder

Bupropion XL (Wellbutrin), bupropion and naltrexone (Revia/Vivitrol) combinations, topiramate (Topamax), and mirtazapine (Remeron) each have some usefulness in treating problematic methamphetamine use.

Bupropion XL (Wellbutrin XL) alone is ineffective at treating daily heavy methamphetamine use, but may have some efficacy in reducing meth use with mild to moderate use of less than 18 days per month. It should be given extra consideration for patients with cooccurring depression and tobacco use disorder. Combined bupropion XL 450 mg daily and naltrexone (Revia, Vivitrol) can help reduce methamphetamine use for moderate to severe methamphetamine use disorder. In the street medicine setting, most clinicians prefer to combine bupropion XL with extended-release injectable naltrexone (Vivitrol). For people with cooccurring OUD, the ASAM/AAAP guidelines recommend this combination of medication only if the person with OUD is already prescribed naltrexone. The bupropion XL and naltrexone combination treatment should be considered for people with cooccurring alcohol and/or tobacco use disorders. See Chap. 4, Sect. 4.6 for prescribing information for bupropion XL and Table 6.3 in this chapter for oral and injectable naltrexone prescribing.

Mirtazapine (Remeron) is less effective than other treatments for methamphetamine use disorder, only showing a small reduction in meth use in placebo-controlled trials. It does appear to significantly reduce sexual risk behaviors and improves sleep quality. Prescribing information for mirtazapine can be found in Chap. 4, Sect. 4.6.

Evidence for topiramate demonstrates its ability to significantly reduce methamphetamine use, though it has poor outcomes with abstinence. Because of cognitive problems and appetite suppression with topiramate, its usefulness in the street medicine setting is limited. However, it may be considered among people with as history of seizures, anorexia, or bulimia given contraindications with bupropion for these disorders. It can also help treat alcohol use disorder.

6.9.4.2 Stimulant Medications for Methamphetamine Use Disorder

The only stimulant medication recommended for methamphetamine use disorder treatment per ASAM/AAAP guidelines is methylphenidate. In their guideline supplement ASAM and AAAP found that prescription amphetamine trials for amphetamine-type stimulant use disorder were plagued by insufficient doses of prescription amphetamines and high drop-out rates. They reference research findings that high doses of prescription stimulants are required for any effectiveness with stimulant use disorders. A high-quality meta-analysis did not show significant improvement in abstinence overall, but higher doses were associated with short-term abstinence. Methylphenidate may also help patients reduce overall use and cravings for methamphetamine. The guidelines suggested additional consideration for methylphenidate treatment for cooccurring ADHD and methamphetamine use disorder. Maximum doses of long-acting methylphenidate products may be most helpful.

Notably, a Swedish nationwide cohort study published in 2022 reported that lisdexamphetamine (Vyvanse) treatment was significantly associated with reduced hospitalizations due to substance use disorder, any hospitalizations or death, and all-cause mortality among people with amphetamine and methamphetamine use disorder, suggesting that randomized controlled trials should be performed looking at lisdexamphetamine as a harm reduction option. The study authors note that there were significant limitations of the study, including that they were unable to determine if lisdexamphetamine was prescribed for ADHD diagnoses or off-label as a treatment of methamphetamine use disorder [31]. ADHD itself is associated with hospitalization and early death, particularly if untreated. The findings of this study could reflect that people with ADHD who were treated with lisdexamphetamine had reduced hospitalizations and mortality because the medication improved ADHD symptoms, not because it reduced the negative impacts of methamphetamine use.

6.10 Opioids

The opioid crisis in North America started by widespread prescribing of opiates for pain relief in the 1990s and 2000s. As people became addicted to prescription opioids the "heroin market" responded to increased demand by supplying synthetic opioids such as fentanyl which is far more potent that prescribed opiates. The more potent synthetic opiates combined with an increasingly toxic drug supply has resulted in an epidemic of opioid overdose deaths. In 2022 there were 7537 deaths due to opioid overdoses in Canada (a rate of 19 deaths per 100,000 which is nearly twice the Canadian suicide rate) and 81,806 opioid overdose deaths in the USA. Heroin and fentanyl predominate among opioids used on the streets, though other synthetic opioids pop up and spread in various geographic areas at times. Counterfeit pills sold as prescription opioids on the streets commonly contain fentanyl and adulterants that are pressed to appear like prescription pharmaceuticals. Counterfeit pills sold as prescription benzodiazepines and stimulants also often contain fentanyl. The majority of street medicine clinicians interviewed for this chapter reported that most patients either inject or smoke opioids, though some occasionally snorting them.

Happiness, relaxation, and pain relief are the primary desired effects for people using opioids. Signs of intoxication with opioids include euphoria, calmness, bradycardia, hypotension, miosis (pinpoint pupils), sedation, slowed movements, and slurred speech. Unpleasant effects include constipation, nausea, vomiting, headache dizziness, sedation, and sleep problems. Opioids can slow the heart rate, lower blood pressure, and cause heart failure and cardiac arrest system. High-dose longer-term opioid use causes people to be more sensitive to pain. Opioids can increase risk for infection by impairing the immune and are associated with depression, psychosis, and sexual dysfunction [32]. Injection opioid use can lead to soft tissue infections, abscesses, and endocarditis.

6.10.1 Reducing Harm from Opioid Use

Safe use supplies are an important component of harm reduction and are the same as supplies used to snort, smoke, or inject cocaine, except that hammer pipes can be used to smoke opioids. A hammer pipe has a Pyrex stem attached to a wider open Pyrex cylinder. When hammer pipes are distributed with safe injecting supplies to people who exclusively inject opioids, they inject less often [33]. Fentanyl test strips help users identify fentanyl in their drugs in areas where heroin still predominates the opioid supply. While most people will still use their heroin if it contains fentanyl, they often use in a safer way, such as using smaller amounts at a time and not using alone. Xylazine test strips also help people use fentanyl more safely.

6.10.2 Responding to an Opioid Overdose

Respiratory depression and hypoxia, central nervous system impairment (lethargy or unconsciousness), and miosis are the hallmarks of opioid overdose. Respirations start as slow and shallow and may decrease to only a few times per minute or cease. Dyspnea, wheezing, and frothy sputum production may also occur. Bradycardia and moderate to severe hypotension occur as well as possible seizures. Clammy or bluish skin is common, though some people may have skin flushing or urticaria due to release of histamine during overdose [34]. Death typically occurs over one to three hours after last injection of fentanyl, though it can feel faster with delays in recognition of overdose.

Compassionate response to overdose encompasses actions and language used during and after the overdose and can very effectively build trust among people sleeping rough. The level of compassion street medicine teams employ impact the willingness of both observers and the person who overdosed to engage with you in the future. Information found online about responding to an opioid overdose instructs responders to call 911. People who use or who have used opioids, harm reduction workers, and seasoned street outreach/ street medicine clinicians express caution or outright opposition to calling emergency responders given both the stigma and discrimination towards people who use drugs and real potential for arrest from police officers responding. A 2017 study described concern of arrest for the homeless victim and witnesses for outstanding warrants as the primary reason for not calling 911. Fears were based on the city's aggressive approach in managing homelessness, including anti-camping bans. Housed people who use drugs were additionally concerned that they would lose their public housing. Good Samaritan laws were insufficient to allay fears [35]. Further, people sleeping rough have been traumatized by experiences with law enforcement and incarceration and do not want to call emergency responders to their camps, whether they are experiencing or witnessing the overdose. Building and maintaining trust with street medicine patients throughout an overdose can be challenging regardless of decisions made or events that occur. Advanced planning within street medicine teams for what to do in the event of an overdose can prepare team members to act rapidly without having the burden of making difficult medical and ethical decisions in an overdose situation.

Regardless of whether you call 911, rapid naloxone (Narcan) administration is important, particularly when the person is unresponsive. Naloxone, an opioid antagonist that reverses opioid overdoses, is available as a spray given intranasally (IN) and a liquid solution that can be injected subcutaneously (SQ) and intramuscularly (IM). If the person is responsive and can look at you, no naloxone is needed yet; stay with them and reassess every two minutes. Monitor with a pulse oximeter if available. If the person becomes unconscious, give naloxone. If you do not have naloxone, call to others for help and ask for naloxone, call 911 if no naloxone is readily available, and perform rescue breathing.

People who use opioids want responders to know, however, the importance of giving the lowest dose of naloxone needed. Recommendations published in 2024 by a panel of harm reduction and lived experience experts note that high doses of naloxone causing painful protracted precipitated withdrawal that are perceived as punitive when administered by medical personnel and law enforcement and fear of punishment results in reduced use of necessary emergency interventions. These experts recommend using doses of 2 mg IN or 0.4 mg IM initially. Naloxone vials typically come with several milliliters of 0.4 mg/mL. Giving higher doses or frequent subsequent doses does not reverse the overdose faster. If after three minutes, the person does not respond to attempts to arouse, have cyanosis or ashen skin, or who are not breathing faster than one respiration every five seconds, give a second dose of naloxone 2 mg IN or 0.4 mg IM. If they do respond, stay with them and continue to monitor [36].

With continued nonresponse after another three minutes, additional doses may be necessary. Some street medicine clinicians have needed doses of 8–12 mg, particularly if carfentanil—a synthetic opioid approximately 100 times more potent than fentanyl—is involved. For individuals who are not breathing, give rescue breathing before and after each dose of naloxone. Using a pulse oximeter can be helpful in monitoring response to naloxone during rescue. With newer veterinary tranquilizer adulterants, such as xylazine and medetomidine, in the fentanyl supply, people who overdose many not have improvement in respiratory depression with naloxone and continued rescue breathing is necessary. See Sect. 6.12 of this chapter for more information about veterinary tranqulizers.

Naloxone reverses the overdose only for 20–90 minutes. If the person does not go to the emergency room after overdose, they need someone to stay with them—either friends on the streets or someone else—to monitor for subsequent need for naloxone or other intervention. The half-life for fentanyl is three to seven hours [37]. Regardless of the amount of naloxone you give, be prepared for a variety of responses by the person who overdosed once they do respond. Some people, even if given the lowest possible dose of naloxone will experience precipitated withdrawal and will respond angrily or aggressively.

Regardless of the amount of experience someone has in managing overdoses in clinical settings, responding to an overdose in the street setting is different. Even if you have reversed many overdoses, be prepared for your own response after reversing an overdose in the street medicine setting. Often, responders feel a mix of emotions: pride, empowerment, overwhelm, anger, sadness, exhilaration, uncertainty, and exhaustion are all normal. Processing your emotional and physical reactions individually and with your team members is important in the aftermath of an overdose. People who have reversed numerous street-based overdoses can also experience these emotions, particularly with unexpected outcomes, unusual circumstances, and if the person overdosing dies.

6.10.3 Management of Opioid Withdrawal

Most—if not all—street medicine patients who use opioids have experienced withdrawal and will do whatever possible to avoid it. Opioid withdrawal is a potentially life-threatening condition, marked by tachycardia, hypertension, possible hyperthermia, insomnia, enlarged pupils, hyperreflexia, sweating, gooseflesh, increased respiratory rate, yawning, runny nose, tearing eyes, muscle spasms, nausea, vomiting, diarrhea, anxiety or irritability, arthralgias, and myalgias. Hyponatremia with protracted vomiting and diarrhea can lead to seizures and death. Aspiration of vomit is another complication from opioid withdrawal. Withdrawal experiences make it difficult to initiate treatment for opioid use disorder and good management of withdrawal is important in building and maintaining trust with your patients.

Patients who are starting medication to treat OUD often successfully complete street-based inductions without significant withdrawal. With buprenorphine, patients need to be in mild withdrawal prior to taking their first dose, typically 12 or more hours after their last use. Methadone does not require stopping opioids prior to starting. Most street medicine teams caution patients not to start naltrexone as their first plan for stopping opioids. Patients need to abstain from opioid use for two weeks prior to starting naltrexone and few are able to undergo withdrawal and abstinence for that duration. Often, however, street medicine patients who have been incarcerated and abstinent for several weeks or longer want to start extended-release injectable naltrexone (Vivitrol) before release from jail or immediately after release from jail.

Some patients may prefer hospitalization for withdrawal management, as methadone can be given IV in that setting. Obstetricians and addiction medicine specialists typically prefer for to manage transition to methadone or buprenorphine among pregnant women in the hospital setting to better prevent withdrawal symptoms, as it adversely affects the fetus. Street medicine patients typically prefer medical respite units as a more compassionate and comfortable place than the hospital if they need or want a supervised transition to buprenorphine. For more information about medical respite, search for Respite Care Providers' Network (RCPN) affiliated with National Health Care for the Homeless Council.

Most street medicine clinicians interviewed for this chapter had similar strategies for preemptive withdrawal management for patients doing street-inductions on buprenorphine. One reported, "I'm willing to give [patients] almost anything for a week" to manage withdrawal. Others were less comfortable with gabapentin and benzodiazepine prescriptions. See the next section on buprenorphine treatment for medications used to manage opioid withdrawal.

6.10.4 Medication Treatment for Opioid Use Disorder

Street-based treatment of opioid use disorder is now common among street medicine teams and successes with buprenorphine have been documented in the literature [38, 39]. On the streets, clinicians typically prescribe buprenorphine (Suboxone, Subutex, Sublocade, Brixadi). Fewer prescribe naltrexone (Revia, Vivtrol) products for OUD, though most will caution against transitioning from heroin or fentanyl straight to naltrexone for reasons described in the last section. In addition, naltrexone is an opioid receptor antagonist, completely blocking the mu opioid receptor. With this blockade, patients are unable to maintain or develop any tolerance to opioids, and are at higher risk of fatal overdose if they miss or stop taking naltrexone. Because patient choice is a vital component of street medicine work and recovery, clinicians should provide the option of naltrexone, as long as patients are able to provide true informed consent about the overdose risk with the medication.

Methadone treatment for OUD remains highly restricted in the United States and can only be prescribed at authorized methadone clinics. Mobile methadone units do exist, but relatively few US street medicine programs offer mobile methadone treatment because of the burden of legal restrictions and requirements. Street medicine clinicians discuss the benefits of methadone with patients, particularly if the person is not ready to stop using opioids, has had a lot of difficulty with withdrawal, has had difficulty with cravings on buprenorphine, or needs more pain control than buprenorphine can offer. Cities usually have multiple methadone programs, though they vary in levels of compassion, punitive rules, and ease of use and access. Rural areas in the U.S. may not have any methadone options. Patients who dislike methadone typically dislike the treatment requirements of having to attend clinic daily and spending half the day traveling, obtaining their dose, and attending any required therapy. Some programs, especially before the covid-19 pandemic, have stringent lengthy requirements of daily attendance and negative urine toxicology prior to allowing patients to take away several days, a week, or a month's supply of methadone.

6.10.4.1 Buprenorphine Treatment

Most street medicine teams offer initial buprenorphine prescriptions and unsupervised buprenorphine inductions on the street, though a few teams only offer the first script on the street if attempts to come to clinic have failed. More teams prefer for patients to come to a clinic staffed by street medicine clinicians for subsequent prescriptions, though most are flexible. Clinicians who prefer this model of treatment believe that clinic offers the opportunity for best and most comprehensive care and articulate a justice-based argument that the privacy offered in clinic should not only be available to all people, but prioritized. Some street medicine teams provide all buprenorphine care in the street medicine setting and believe that clinical settings are both too psychologically traumatic and too impractical for their patients. These teams argue that the patient's own environment offers patients the most autonomy, authority, and safety. The geography in which the street medicine team functions more often dictates how services are provided. Teams in small geographic areas with numerous small clinical spaces in shelters and other homeless services organizations tend to prefer the clinic-based approach. Almost all teams had the ability to offer in-clinic buprenorphine induction for patients who had difficulty inducting on their own or the rare patient who preferred a clinic-based induction.

Buprenorphine induction is typically accomplished with micro-dosing, low-dose, or high-dose inductions. While most street clinicians have some preference or comfort with one over the other, but most follow what one clinician described as "buyer's choice." Not all low- and high-dose inductions are alike, though most follow a similar strategy listed in Table 6.5. The only clinician who reported micro-dosing noted that nearly all patients were smoking fentanyl, not injecting.

Concomitantly with initial prescriptions for buprenorphine, most clinicians give comfort medications. Most teams provide medications for nausea and vomiting, diarrhea, anxiety, and muscle spasm or pain. Combinations of four to five medications are common. One person noted not including gabapentin for withdrawal management until xylazine and medetomidine infiltrated the fentanyl supply. Gabapentin helps with severe anxiety related to tranquilizer withdrawal. See Table 6.6 for

Table 6.5 Micro-dosing, low-, and high-dose inductions on buprenorphine

Type of induction	Timing of initial dose	Amount of initial dose	Next dose	Total in first 24 hours	Usual maintenance dose
High-dose	10–20 hours after last use	8 mg at once	Second 8 mg whenever withdrawal symptoms occur or in 8 hours	24 mg	24 to 32 mg daily divided BID or TID
Low-dose	10–12 hours after last use	1–2 mg or a small bite off a film	Next dose in ½ -1 hour if no withdrawal or in 2 hours if withdrawal symptoms occur	16 mg; take bites or 1–2 mg dose up to 8 mg in the first 12 hours, then 8 mg 12 hours later	16–24 mg daily divided BID or TID.
Micro-dosing	When in mild withdrawal	0.5 mg only on first day	Increase by 0.5 mg daily for 6–7 days	n/a	8 mg BID

Table 6.6 Comfort medications for opioid withdrawal

Symptom(s) treated	Common medications	Less common medications
Nausea, vomiting	Odansetron (Zofran) 4 mg PRN Q6h	
Diarrhea	Loperamide (Imodium) 2 mg PRN each loose stool. Max dose 8 mg /24 hours	
Anxiety	Clonidine (Catapres) 0.1 mg Q8h PRN Gabapentin (Neurontin) 300 mg BID Hydroxyzine pamoate (Vistaril) 25–50 mg Q 6 h prn	Clonazepam (Klonopin) 0.5–1 mg po BID Lorazepam (Ativan) 0.5-1 mg BID or TID
Pain, muscle spasm	Tylenol 1000 mg BID Methocarbamol 500 mg Q6h PRN	Ibuprofen (Motrin) 600 mg Q6h PRN

comfort medications and doses. Typically, clinicians give at least two or three anxiety medications listed. One team starts clonidine transdermal patch (Catapres-TTS) 0.1 mg three weeks prior to induction, then increases by 0.1 mg each week, and continues it for several weeks after induction. This team treats many patients with severe anxiety disorders.

One street psychiatrist reported a very high success rate of induction using high-dose induction and long-acting injectable buprenorphine (Sublocade) 300 mg within the first week. They found that most patients remained on the long-acting injection, but preferred to continue to have access to some sublingual buprenorphine at the same time. The patients treated by this team all have serious mental illness and many were already taking long-acting injectable antipsychotics when the injectable buprenorphine was started. Most teams start patients on injectable buprenorphine whenever they were ready and have low interest from most patients currently sleeping rough. They do see more interest among patients once they move into housing. At the time of interview, no teams were using the brand name buprenorphine injection, Brixadi, for street medicine patients. One clinician noted that Brixadi is easier to start, but Sublocade was more effective for patients.

Some teams give one-week prescriptions at the time of induction and others give enough for several days, then check in with the patient to prescribe more. One clinician gave an initial two- to four-week supply of buprenorphine due to the team's inability to connect with patients more frequently.

6.11 Psychedelics

MDMA (Ecstasy), psilocybin, mescaline (peyote), LSD, PCP, ayahuasca, and other numerous other drugs can be classified as psychedelics/ hallucinogens. Street medicine team may find patients use them more in certain geographic locations than others, but they are less commonly used among people sleeping rough in North America today. Clinicians working with First Nation and Inuit people report that mescaline and ayahuasca are used ceremonially, but are overused among people indigenous to North America. These drugs typically have desired effects of euphoria, feelings of social connectedness and deeper understanding of oneself, and dissociation. Most psychedelics can cause elevated blood pressure, tachycardia, elevated body temperature, and memory problems with regular use. Toxicity can lead to seizures, coma, and death. If use of any of these substances is common in your street medicine patient population, read additional information online and in medical journals. Treatment strategies are all psychosocial interventions, as medication treatments do not exist. Some psychedelics are used to treat substance use disorders.

6.12 Synthetic Cathinones (Bath Salts)

Typically swallowed, sniffed, snorted, or injected, synthetic cathinones are human-made stimulants that are chemically similar to cathinones in the khat plant, a shrub grown in East Africa and southern Arabia [40]. They cause alertness, euphoria, increased sociability, and increased sex drive similar to cocaine, methamphetamine, and MDMA (ecstasy) and are legally marketed in the United States as "research chemicals," "glass cleaners," and "bath salts" and labeled "not meant for human consumption." Because producers can slightly alter chemical structure of each synthetic cathinone while maintaining the overall stimulant effect, governments attempting to ban each substance have difficulty keeping up.

6.12.1 Synthetic Cathinone Intoxication and Withdrawal

Aside from the desired effects, bath salts produce a host of undesirable effects including hypertension, tachycardia, dilated pupils, sweating, headaches, nausea, vomiting, confusion, agitation, aggressive or violent behavior, paranoia, hallucinations, panic attacks, insomnia, and suicidal thoughts. Choreathetosis, involuntary movements characterized by a combination of rapid, jerky, and irregular movements (chorea) and slow, writhing movements (athetosis), can be observed during intoxication and beyond [41]. Overdose produces a sympathomimetic toxidrome, like cocaine and methamphetamine, that includes autonomic instability, seizures, and rhabdomyolysis. When severe, the toxidrome leads to kidney failure, coronary and cerebral ischemia, hyperthermia, intracranial hemorrhage, cardiovascular collapse, and death. Withdrawal symptoms include depression, poor energy and motivation, and drug cravings [42].

Treatments are typically supportive and may include benzodiazepines and antipsychotics in emergency room and hospital settings with overdose. There are no medications used to treat synthetic cathinone use disorder at this time. Off-label treatments for other stimulant use disorders, such as combination injectable naltrexone and bupropion, topiramate, and prescriptions stimulants have not been evaluated for bath salts. Interestingly, bupropion itself is a synthetic cathinone.

6.13 Tranquilizers

Though some regions in North America have yet to see them, xylazine (tranq) and medetomidine are veterinary tranquilizers that are increasingly implicated in overdose deaths in North America. In the United States, xylazine-positive over dose deaths increase by over 100% in all regions and an impressive 1127% in the South [43]. Xylazine was first discovered as an adulterant in the drug supply in 2015 and medetomidine in 2022 [44]. Primarily mixed with fentanyl, both xylazine and medetomidine cause severe respiratory depression and do not respond to naloxone (Narcan). As central nervous system depressants, they also cause sedation, muscle relaxation, dangerously low blood pressure, bradycardia, seizures, and death. Seizures are more prominent with medetomidine than with xylazine. Both cause vasoconstriction, which is thought to be the pathophysiology of xylazine wounds and explains why the wounds occur whether xylazine is injected or swallowed in a counterfeit pill. Medetomidine does not cause substantial wounds, but its vasoconstriction does cause falsely low pulse oximetry results, muscle twitching, and hypothermia. Seizures are more common with medetomidine. Withdrawal can cause crippling anxiety as well as hypertension, tachycardia, nausea, vomiting, insomnia, restlessness, and dizziness. Clonidine is thought to be helpful in withdrawal management, but patients should be closely monitored for hypotension [45]. Xylazine has been found in cocaine, K2, and other drugs. Most people are accidentally using these tranquilizers. Harm reduction includes xylazine test strips, early detection and treatment of wounds, and teaching drug users to care for their own and others' xylazine wounds.

6.14 Tobacco

Tobacco use disorder receives little attention from the street medicine community, though it contributes to nearly a fifth of early deaths among people who are homeless [46]. In fact, approximately 15% of homeless health care providers distribute cigarettes in an effort to build trust [47]. While tobacco use is declining in North America, nearly 75% of people who are homeless smoke cigarettes, 4 times higher than the U.S. adult population and 2.5 times higher than Americans living in poverty [48]. No information about tobacco use disorder or its health impacts in unsheltered populations. Clinicians interviewed for this chapter reported wide variations in tobacco use among their patients, with some seeing very few patients who smoke and others reporting near universal use among patients.

6.14.1 Reducing Harm from Tobacco Use

Many people living unsheltered cannot afford cigarettes and either share with others or buy loose tobacco to roll their own. Sniping, or smoking the butts of cigarettes in used ashtrays is common, particularly among homeless youth [49]. Cigarette filters in public ashtrays provide an excellent medium for growing bacteria and other pathogens. Street medicine teams can reduce harm by providing rolling papers to encourage patients who snipe to remove the tobacco from sniped cigarettes and roll their own cigarettes. Rolling paper packages are about a quarter to a third of the cost of a pack of cigarettes and contain 32 papers. For people who have health insurance and do not want to stop using nicotine, consider prescribing ongoing nicotine replacement products. Nicotine gum, lozenges, and patches provide safer options for nicotine consumption compared to chewing tobacco and cigarettes. Encourage patients who have vape pens to only use tobacco in their cartridges.

6.14.2 Medication Treatment for Tobacco Use Disorder

Prescribe Varenicline (Chantix), bupropion XL (Wellbutrin XL), bupropion SR (Zyban), or nicotine replacement products for people who want to cut back or quit smoking. See Table 6.7 for information on nicotine replacement prescribing. Nicotine replacement therapies may be combined if needed. Instruct patients to stop using other tobacco products when they start replacement therapy. Patches are longer-acting and can be prescribed with the short-acting products (gum, lozenges, spray, and inhaler). The spray offers the fastest nicotine delivery and the lozenges provide about 25% more nicotine than the gum [50].

Both varenicline (Chantix) and bupropion (Wellbutrin, Zyban) help people quit smoking, but varenicline is superior to bupropion in promoting abstinence [51]. Varenicline is typically well-tolerated, but can cause sore throat, stuffy nose, diarrhea, heartburn, insomnia, dizziness, and has a bad taste. It does not cause seizures and is a safer option on the streets. It is dosed twice daily compared to bupropion

Table 6.7 Nicotine replacement therapy

Product	Dose	Instructions
Patches	7 mg if <5 cig/day 14 mg if 6–10 cig/day 21 mg if >10 cig/day	Change patch daily. Use for 6 to 12 weeks, tapering dose over time. Stop patches when ready.
Gum	Use 2 mg if time of first cigarette is >30 minutes after waking and for <20 cig/day. Use 4 mg if time of first cigarette is <30 minutes after waking and for >20 cig/day	Use 1 piece Q1-2h PRN, max 20 per day. Chew until peppery taste or tingling in mouth occurs, then tuck in cheek. Chew again when taste or tingling disappears. Each piece of gum lasts 30 minutes. Taper over time as tolerated.
Lozenges	Same dosing instructions as gum	Use 1 lozenge Q1-2h PRN, max 24 per day. Place in between cheek and gums. Do not chew, suck, or swallow. Taper over time as tolerated.
Inhaler	10 mg/cartridge = 4 mg nicotine. Each cartridge contains 80 sips	Use 1 cartridge Q1-2h PRN, max 16 per day. Sip like a drink rather than using like an inhaler. Taper over time as tolerated.
Spray	10 mg/mL. Each bottle contains 200 sprays.	1 spray in each nostril Q1h or as needed. Taper over time as tolerated.

Table 6.8 Medications for smoking cessation

Medication	Initial dose	Next dose	Next dose	Other
Bupropion XL (Wellbutrin XL)	150 mg Qam × 3 days	300 mg Qam	Not applicable	Take at least 12 weeks, but may continue beyond
Varenicline (Chantix)	0.5 mg Qam on day 1	0.5 mg BID on days 4–7	1 mg BID on day 8 and beyond	Take for 8 to 35 days

XL, which is dosed once daily. The FDA removed its black box warning on varenicline in 2016, as it was found not to significantly contribute to suicidal ideation [52]. See Table 6.8 for varenicline and bupropion XL dosing for smoking cessation. Both medications should be taken for a week before the patient tries to quit. Though the brand name bupropion SR (Zyban) is marketed for smoking cessation, the XL formulation can be given once daily and is easier to use in the street medicine setting.

References

1. Podymow T, Turnbull J, Coyle D, Yetisir E, Wells G. Shelter-based managed alcohol administration to chronically homeless people addicted to alcohol. CMAJ. 2006;174(1):45.
2. Montgomery AE, Szymkowiak D, Marcus J, Howard P, Culhane DP. Homelessness, Unsheltered status, and risk factors for mortality: findings from the 100 000 homes campaign. Public Health Rep [Internet]. 2016 1 [cited 2025 May 8];131(6):765. Available from: https://pmc.ncbi.nlm.nih.gov/articles/PMC5230839/
3. Roncarati JS, Baggett TP, O'Connell JJ, Hwang SW, Francis Cook E, Krieger N, et al. Mortality among unsheltered homeless adults in Boston, Massachusetts, 2000–2009. JAMA Intern Med [Internet]. 2018 [cited 2025 May 8];178(9):1242. Available from: https://pmc.ncbi.nlm.nih.gov/articles/PMC6142967/
4. Motta-Ochoa R, Incio-Serra N, Brulotte A, Flores-Aranda J. Motives for alcohol use, risky drinking patterns and harm reduction practices among people who experience homelessness and alcohol dependence in Montreal. Harm Reduct J [Internet]. 2023 [cited 2025 May 8];20(1):1–12. Available from: https://harmreductionjournal.biomedcentral.com/articles/10.1186/s12954-023-00757-2
5. Collins SE. Harm reduction treatment for substance use: meeting people where they're at. [PowerPoint presentation]. Harm Reduction Research and Treatment Center, University of Washington. [cited 2025 May 8]; Available from: http://www.adcouncil.org
6. Harm Reduction Strategies for Alcohol – Partnership to End Addiction [Internet]. [cited 2025 May 9]. Available from: https://drugfree.org/article/harm-reduction-strategies-for-alcohol/
7. Smith-Bernardin SM, Suen LW, Barr-Walker J, Cuervo IA, Handley MA. Scoping review of managed alcohol programs. Harm Reduct J [Internet]. 2022 Dec 1 [cited 2025 May 9];19(1):1–27. Available from: https://harmreductionjournal.biomedcentral.com/articles/10.1186/s12954-022-00646-0
8. Interrupted Memories: Alcohol-Induced Blackouts | National Institute on Alcohol Abuse and Alcoholism (NIAAA) [Internet]. [cited 2025 May 9]. Available from: https://www.niaaa.nih.gov/publications/brochures-and-fact-sheets/interrupted-memories-alcohol-induced-blackouts
9. Bayard M, Mcintyre J, Hill KR, Jack Woodside J. Alcohol withdrawal syndrome. Am Fam Physician [Internet] 2004 [cited 2025 May 9];69(6):1443–1450. Available from: https://www.aafp.org/pubs/afp/issues/2004/0315/p1443.html
10. Maldonado JR, Sher Y, Das S, Hills-Evans K, Frenklach A, Lolak S, et al. Prospective validation study of the prediction of alcohol withdrawal severity scale (PAWSS) in medically

ill inpatients: a new scale for the prediction of complicated alcohol withdrawal syndrome. Alcohol Alcoholism [Internet] 2015 [cited 2025 May 9];50(5):509–518. Available from: https://pubmed.ncbi.nlm.nih.gov/25999438/
11. Maisel NC, Blodgett JC, Wilbourne PL, Humphreys K, Finney JW. Meta-analysis of naltrexone and acamprosate for treating alcohol use disorders: when are these medications most helpful? Addiction (Abingdon, England) [Internet]. 2012 [cited 2025 May 9];108(2):275. Available from: https://pmc.ncbi.nlm.nih.gov/articles/PMC3970823/
12. McPheeters M, O'Connor EA, Riley S, Kennedy SM, Voisin C, Kuznacic K, et al. Pharmacotherapy for alcohol use disorder: a systematic review and meta-analysis. JAMA [Internet]. 2023 [cited 2025 May 9];330(17):1653–65. Available from: https://jamanetwork.com/journals/jama/fullarticle/2811435
13. Kalk NJ, Lingford-Hughes AR. The clinical pharmacology of acamprosate. Br J Clin Pharmacol [Internet] 2014 [cited 2025 May 9];77(2):315. Available from: https://pmc.ncbi.nlm.nih.gov/articles/PMC4014018/
14. Disulfiram (oral route) – Mayo Clinic [Internet]. [cited 2025 May 9]. Available from: https://www.mayoclinic.org/drugs-supplements/disulfiram-oral-route/description/drg-20063488
15. Edinoff AN, Nix CA, Odisho AS, Babin CP, Derouen AG, Lutfallah SC, et al. Novel designer benzodiazepines: comprehensive review of evolving clinical and adverse effects. Neurol Int. 2022;14:648–663 [Internet]. 2022 [cited 2025 May 9];14(3):648–63. Available from: https://www.mdpi.com/2035-8377/14/3/53/htm
16. https://www.canada.ca/en/health-canada/services/opioids/responding-canada-opioid-crisis/safer-supply.html [Internet]. 2023. Safer Supply.
17. Benzodiazepine overdose – Symptoms, diagnosis and treatment | BMJ Best Practice US [Internet]. [cited 2025 May 9]. Available from: https://bestpractice.bmj.com/topics/en-us/343
18. Hood SD, Norman A, Hince DA, Melichar JK, Hulse GK. Benzodiazepine dependence and its treatment with low dose flumazenil. Br J Clin Pharmacol [Internet]. 2014 Feb [cited 2025 May 9];77(2):285. Available from: https://pmc.ncbi.nlm.nih.gov/articles/PMC4014019/
19. Coombs T, Abdelkader A, Ginige T, Van Calster P, Harper M, Al-Jumeily D, et al. Understanding drug use patterns among the homeless population: a systematic review of quantitative studies. Emerging Trends Drugs Addict Health [Internet]. 2024 [cited 2025 May 9];4:100059. Available from: https://www.sciencedirect.com/science/article/pii/S2667118223000107
20. Richards J, Kuhn R. Unsheltered homelessness and health: a literature review. AJPM Focus [Internet]. 2022 [cited 2025 May 9];2(1):100043. Available from: https://pmc.ncbi.nlm.nih.gov/articles/PMC10546518/
21. Brousseau VD, Bahl E, Lacroix-Labonté J, Robichaud A, Lefsrud M. Fungal contamination monitoring in legal cannabis using ultra-high performance liquid chromatography tandem mass spectrometry. J Test Eval. 2024;52(6):3165.
22. Gagnon M, McRitchie T, Montsion K, Tully J, Blais M, Snider N, et al. High levels of pesticides found in illicit cannabis inflorescence compared to licensed samples in Canadian study using expanded 327 pesticides multiresidue method. J Cannabis Res. 2023;5(1):34.
23. Outbreak of Lung Injury Associated with the Use of E-Cigarette, or Vaping, Products | CDC Archive [Internet]. [cited 2025 May 9]. Available from: https://archive.cdc.gov/#/details?url=https://www.cdc.gov/tobacco/basic_information/e-cigarettes/severe-lung-disease.html
24. Drugs A to Z | National Institute on Drug Abuse (NIDA) [Internet]. [cited 2025 May 9]. Available from: https://nida.nih.gov/research-topics/drugs-a-to-z#cannabis
25. Marijuana (Weed) Withdrawal: Symptoms & Treatment [Internet]. [cited 2025 May 9]. Available from: https://my.clevelandclinic.org/health/diseases/marijuana-weed-withdrawal
26. Coombs T, Ginige T, Van Calster P, Abdelkader A, Corazza O, Assi S. New psychoactive substances in the homeless population: a cross-sectional study in the United Kingdom. Int J Ment Health Addict [Internet] 2024 [cited 2025 May 9];22(4):2322–2337. Available from: https://link.springer.com/article/10.1007/s11469-022-00988-7
27. de Oliveira MC, Vides MC, Lassi DLS, Torales J, Ventriglio A, Bombana HS, et al. Toxicity of synthetic cannabinoids in K2/spice: a systematic review. Brain Sci [Internet] 2023 [cited 2025 May 9];13(7):990. Available from: https://pmc.ncbi.nlm.nih.gov/articles/PMC10377539/

28. The ASAM/AAAP clinical practice guideline on the management of stimulant use disorder. J Addict Med [Internet] 2024 [cited 2025 May 9];18(1):1–56. Available from: https://journals.lww.com/journaladdictionmedicine/fulltext/2024/05001/the_asam_aaap_clinical_practice_guideline_on_the.1.aspx
29. Lavonas EJ, Akpunonu PD, Arens AM, Babu KM, Cao D, Hoffman RS, et al. 2023 American Heart Association focused update on the Management of Patients with Cardiac Arrest or life-threatening toxicity due to poisoning: an update to the American Heart Association guidelines for cardiopulmonary resuscitation and emergency cardiovascular care. Circulation. 2023;148(16):E149–84.
30. Acheson LS, Williams BH, Farrell M, McKetin R, Ezard N, Siefried KJ. Pharmacological treatment for methamphetamine withdrawal: a systematic review and meta-analysis of randomised controlled trials. Drug Alcohol Rev [Internet] 2022 [cited 2025 May 9];42(1):7. Available from: https://pmc.ncbi.nlm.nih.gov/articles/PMC10083934/
31. Heikkinen M, Taipale H, Tanskanen A, Mittendorfer-Rutz E, Lähteenvuo M, Tiihonen J. Association of Pharmacological Treatments and Hospitalization and death in individuals with amphetamine use disorders in a Swedish Nationwide cohort of 13 965 patients. JAMA Psychiatry [Internet] 2023 [cited 2025 May 9];80(1):31–9. Available from: https://jamanetwork.com/journals/jamapsychiatry/fullarticle/2798882
32. Pathan H, Williams J. Basic opioid pharmacology: an update. Br J Pain. 2012;6(1):11–6.
33. Fitzpatrick T, McMahan VM, Frank ND, Glick SN, Violette LR, Davis S, et al. Heroin pipe distribution to reduce high-risk drug consumption behaviors among people who use heroin: a pilot quasi-experimental study. Harm Reduct J [Internet] 2022 [cited 2025 May 9];19(1):1–14. Available from: https://harmreductionjournal.biomedcentral.com/articles/10.1186/s12954-022-00685-7
34. Regina AC, Goyal A, Mechanic OJ. Opioid toxicity. Challenging cases and complication management in pain medicine [Internet]. 2025 [cited 2025 May 9];3–7. Available from: https://www.ncbi.nlm.nih.gov/books/NBK470415/
35. Koester S, Mueller SR, Raville L, Langegger S, Binswanger IA. Why are some people who have received overdose education and naloxone reticent to call Emergency Medical Services in the event of overdose? Int J Drug Policy [Internet]. 2017 [cited 2025 May 9];48:115. Available from: https://pmc.ncbi.nlm.nih.gov/articles/PMC5825210/
36. Russell E, Hawk M, Neale J, Bennett AS, Davis C, Hill LG, et al. A call for compassionate opioid overdose response. Int J Drug Policy [Internet]. 2024 [cited 2025 May 9];133:104587. Available from: https://www.sciencedirect.com/science/article/pii/S0955395924002718
37. Dunn KE, Bird HE, Durgin CJ. Fentanyl. The Oxford handbook of opioids and opioid use disorder [Internet]. 2023 [cited 2025 May 9];317–53. Available from: https://www.ncbi.nlm.nih.gov/books/NBK459275/
38. Carter J, Zevin B, Lum PJ. Low barrier buprenorphine treatment for persons experiencing homelessness and injecting heroin in San Francisco. Addict Sci Clin Pract [Internet] 2019 [cited 2025 May 9];14(1):20. Available from: https://pmc.ncbi.nlm.nih.gov/articles/PMC6501460/
39. Gibson CL, Lo E. Low-Barrier buprenorphine treatment for people experiencing homelessness. Psychiatr Serv [Internet]. 2023 [cited 2025 May 9];74(1):104. Available from: https://psychiatryonline.org/doi/pdf/10.1176/appi.ps.20220426?download=true
40. Synthetic Cathinones ("Bath Salts") | National Institute on Drug Abuse (NIDA) [Internet]. [cited 2025 May 9]. Available from: https://nida.nih.gov/research-topics/synthetic-cathinones-bath-salts
41. Sutamtewagul G, Sood V, Nugent K. Sympathomimetic syndrome, choreoathetosis, and acute kidney injury following "bath salts" injection. Clin Nephrol [Internet] 2014 [cited 2025 May 9];81(1):63–66. Available from: https://pubmed.ncbi.nlm.nih.gov/24356039/
42. Antoniou T, Juurlink DN. Five things to know about..."bath salts". CMAJ [Internet]. 2012 [cited 2025 May 9];184(15):1713. Available from: https://pmc.ncbi.nlm.nih.gov/articles/PMC3478356/
43. Doj, Dea. DEA joint intelligence report the growing threat of Xylazine and its mixture with illicit drugs. 2022.

44. Fredric Rieders Family Foundation. Toxic adulterant alert: medetomidine/dexmedetomidine. 2023.
45. Franklin F, Teixeira D, Silva DA, Dpa AB. Public health division of substance use prevention and harm reduction • 123 South Broad St, 11th Floor. 1910 [cited 2025 May 9]; Available from: https://www.substanceusephilly.com; https://www.phila.gov/programs/substance-use-prevention-and-harm-reduction; https://hip.phila.gov
46. Baggett TP, Chang Y, Singer DE, Porneala BC, Gaeta JM, O'Connell JJ, et al. Tobacco-, alcohol-, and drug-attributable deaths and their contribution to mortality disparities in a cohort of homeless adults in Boston. Am J Public Health [Internet]. 2015 [cited 2025 May 9];105(6):1189. Available from: https://pmc.ncbi.nlm.nih.gov/articles/PMC4431083/
47. Baggett TP, Anderson R, Freyder PJ, Jarvie JA, Maryman K, Porter J, et al. Addressing tobacco use in homeless populations: a survey of health care professionals. J Health Care Poor Underserved [Internet]. 2012 [cited 2025 May 9];23(4):1650–9. Available from: https://pubmed.ncbi.nlm.nih.gov/23698679/
48. Baggett TP, Tobey ML, Rigotti NA. Tobacco use among homeless people — addressing the neglected addiction. N Engl J Med [Internet] 2013 [cited 2025 May 9];369(3):201–204. Available from: https://www.nejm.org/doi/pdf/10.1056/NEJMp1301935
49. Sniping: Homeless Youths' High-Risk Smoking Practice | RAND [Internet]. [cited 2025 May 9]. Available from: https://www.rand.org/pubs/commentary/2015/10/sniping-homeless-youths-high-risk-smoking-practice.html
50. Tobacco Treatment Medication Dosing Guidelines. 2016.
51. Patel AR, Panchal JR, Desai CK. Efficacy of varenicline versus bupropion for smoking cessation: a systematic review and meta-analysis of randomized controlled trials. Indian J Psychiatry [Internet] 2023 [cited 2025 May 9];65(5):526–533. Available from: https://pubmed.ncbi.nlm.nih.gov/37397838/
52. FDA removes black box warning from Varenicline's label. NEJM J Watch [Internet] 2016 [cited 2025 May 9]. Available from: https://www.jwatch.org/FW112367/2016/12/19/fda-removes-black-box-warning-varenicclines-label

Cognitive Impairment 7

7.1 Prevalence and Recognition

Cognitive impairment among individuals experiencing homelessness is an under-recognized but important health issue. This chapter explores the prevalence, causes, consequences, and service implications of cognitive impairment in people who are homeless.

Cognitive impairment encompasses a broad spectrum of deficits in memory, attention, executive function, and problem solving abilities. Among the general population, mild cognitive impairment and more severe forms such as dementia are typically associated with aging. However, in homeless populations, these impairments are disproportionately common, often affecting younger individuals as well. Studies estimate that between 20% and 80% of people experiencing homelessness exhibit some form of cognitive impairment, depending on the diagnostic criteria and assessment methods used [1–4]. The causes of cognitive impairment in homeless populations include traumatic brain injury, substance abuse, anoxic brain damage due to opioid overdoses, dementia, some mental illnesses, the effects of early life adversity, and developmental disorders. This can have a significant effect on a person's ability to follow instructions, navigate complex health and social systems, problem solve, and organize themselves to stay safe. Also, the experience of being homeless, (for example sleep deprivation), will exacerbate any cognitive impairment, as being homeless you need to have your "wits about you" due to changing environments, institutional demands, and keeping yourself safe.

Despite this high prevalence and serious effects, cognitive impairment often goes undetected and undiagnosed in this population. One reason for under-recognition is the overlapping symptomatology with psychiatric disorders, substance use and the effects of trauma. Additionally, frontline service providers may lack the training or resources to conduct appropriate cognitive screening and helping individuals survive is a priority. Also, individuals themselves may be unaware of or unable to

S. Hatcher et al., *Street Mental Health Handbook*,
https://doi.org/10.1007/978-3-032-00663-9_7

articulate their cognitive difficulties. These challenges are compounded by the chaotic and unstable circumstances of homelessness, which can hide the identification of persistent cognitive deficits [5].

7.2 Etiological Factors

The causes of cognitive impairment among people who are homeless are multifactorial and often overlap.

7.2.1 Traumatic Brain Injury

Traumatic brain injury (TBI) is a major contributor, with prevalence rates in homeless populations substantially higher than in the general public. A systematic review of 38 studies found a lifetime prevalence of any traumatic brain injury in people who are homeless of 53% and moderate to severe injury of 23% [6]. The history of traumatic brain injury was associated with poorer self-reported health, an increase in suicide risk, memory difficulties, and increased health service use and criminal justice system involvement. Traumatic brain injuries may result from physical assaults, falls, accidents, or self-harm and are often unreported or untreated. A more recent report of the prevalence of traumatic brain injury in a population of 127 people experiencing homelessness in California found nearly 80% had a history of traumatic brain injury compared to about 7% in the general population [7]. This is similar to the proportion of 82% reported in a Canadian sample of 285 precariously housed people who also reported that being a victim of an assault was the most common cause [6]. A systematic review of the association between traumatic brain injury and subsequent neurological and psychiatric illness in people experiencing homelessness, found that the odds of someone who was homeless developing a neurological or psychiatric disorder after a traumatic brain injury was about twice that of the housed population [8].

7.2.2 Substance Use

Substance use, particularly chronic alcohol use, is another significant factor. Substances of abuse can have neurotoxic effects, leading to both acute and chronic impairments. Chronic alcohol use can lead to Korsakoff's syndrome caused by Vitamin B1 deficiency which results in difficulty forming new memories and sometimes, making up stories to fill the gap (confabulation). One study in Scotland found that 82% of homeless hostel dwellers had cognitive impairment and one in five had alcohol related brain damage [9]. Hypoxic brain damage following an opioid overdose is becoming increasingly important as a result of the opioid epidemic. A systematic review of 79 articles found evidence of leukoencephalopathy (brain white matter disease) and an "amnestic syndrome" after an opioid overdose [10]. However, the evidence base was weak and the main clinical lesson from the review was the importance of screening people for cognitive impairment after an overdose. Chronic methamphetamine use is associated with cognitive deficits especially in the areas of impulsivity and social cognition [11]. Crack cocaine use affects attention, verbal memory, and learning, which seem to persist at least in the early stages of withdrawal [12].

7.2.3 Dementia

There is evidence that the proportion of unhoused people over the age of 50 is growing rapidly. Recent estimates suggest that 20% of the homeless population in the US is aged 55 and over and of these one in four were unsheltered [13]. The problems of aging while homeless are captured in these quotes from a presentation by Alexis Kogan from the Keck School of Medicine in California.

> "*Well, I realized that being immobile out here is just not an option.*" –Patient
>
> "Sometimes I'm supposed to [take medication] but they make you tired and then what do you do? Or sometimes you can't be in the sun…'Oh, go hang out in the mall for a quick [air conditioning] fix.' Like that's so easy to do; *You're chased constantly. 'You got to go. You can't be here.'*" –Patient
>
> "You also have patients who don't really need a wheelchair for mobility but it's a place they can always sit…and they often choose to sleep (when they do *sleep) sitting up so that they can be more on guard if you get attacked.*" –MD

One study screened all adults 55 and over presenting to a homeless shelter in Phoenix Arizona with the Montreal Cognitive Assessment (MoCA). The authors found 93% of people screened were positive for dementia or mild cognitive impairment using a cutoff of 26 and 72% were positive using a more conservative cut [14]. A population study in Ontario Canada of provincial health service data found that people who were homeless were 1.9 times more likely to have a diagnosis of dementia compared to the general population [15].

7.2.4 Mental Illness

Mental illness, particularly schizophrenia and bipolar disorder, is both a cause and consequence of homelessness and may contribute to cognitive dysfunction. Studies from India have shown that women with schizophrenia who are homeless have significantly greater cognitive impairments than women with schizophrenia living with families [16]. Cognitive deficits in schizophrenia, which are similar to those seen in bipolar disorder, include difficulties with attention, working memory, verbal learning, and executive function. Depression can also cause significant memory issues, which can be mistaken for dementia.

7.2.5 Early Life Adversity and Developmental Disorders

Early-life adversity, including abuse, neglect, and educational disruptions, can result in neurodevelopmental impairments that persist into adulthood such as Fetal Alcohol Syndrome. Developmental disorders with various links to childhood adversity such as Autism Spectrum Disorders, Attention-Deficit/Hyperactivity Disorders, and Learning Disabilities can also contribute to cognitive impairment.

Fetal Alcohol Syndrome Fetal Alcohol Syndrome (FAS) is caused by prenatal alcohol exposure. It leads to a range of physical, cognitive, and behavioral impairments although it is often misdiagnosed and undiagnosed. There is no specific test for it although classically people with fetal alcohol syndrome have characteristic facial features including a thin upper lip, indistinct philtrum (the grooves between nose and upper lip) and short palpebral fissures (the area between open eyelids) as well as impaired growth [17]. Symptoms include poor memory, inattention, learning difficulties, impulsivity and difficulties in social situations. In DSM V the disorder is a "condition under further review" as a Neurobehavioral Disorder associated with prenatal alcohol exposure and includes impaired neurocognitive function, impaired self-regulation and impaired adaptive function. These impairments can significantly affect an individual's ability to navigate life's challenges, increasing the risk of homelessness. There is little information about the proportion of people who are homeless who have fetal alcohol syndrome but most adults with the disorder live or have lived in supported living environments [18]. There is also a clear overlap between the effects of fetal alcohol syndrome, the experience of trauma, substance use and mental disorders. Management focuses on adapting the environment to mitigate the effects of the disorder which includes consistent, stable, and trauma-informed housing and approaches that address the cognitive, mental health, and social needs of people with fetal alcohol syndrome [18].

Autism Spectrum Disorders Autism spectrum disorders affect how someone perceives and socializes with others and may also include limited and repetitive patterns of behavior. Symptoms usually appear in early childhood and can cause difficulties at school. There is limited epidemiological data on the prevalence of autism amongst people who are homeless but one study in London found 12% of a sample of 106 people met DSM V criteria for autism spectrum disorder [19] and another study by the same team in Dublin found a prevalence of 3% [20]. Qualitative studies find the lack of control over routine and environment are particular issues as well as difficulty engaging with services which may not make allowances for the autism diagnosis [21]. Examples are ambient noise when sleeping outside or fluorescent lighting, loud noises and overstimulation when sleeping in shelters. Stone [21] quotes a participant who was unable to do his usual routines and the effect it had on his mental health:

> I couldn't do that [routine] . . . because I didn't know where I was the next day, let alone the next few days . . . I tried laying down on the bench, the wind would blow the leaves across the floor and I am up straight away . . . it brought so much fear into me that even today I still struggle. . . now I am more fearful because of being on the streets and having to have my own back and not knowing what's going to happen from one minute to the next.

Some people with autism respond to stressors with dysregulated emotions and sometimes self-harm, which may cause outreach workers to be afraid of them or want to hospitalize them. Misunderstanding of social cues gives people with autism an extra set of challenges in interacting with homeless support staff who may not recognize autism or know how to help.

Attention-Deficit/Hyperactivity Disorders This is a group of disorders that includes persistent problems with paying attention, impulsivity and, particularly in children, hyperactivity. People with this diagnosis will often have a history of having difficulty at school with paying attention and disciplinary problems. In homeless children and adolescents about a quarter of them will have this diagnosis [22]. There is a strong association between the experience of childhood abuse and the presence of ADHD [23]. However, what is not clear is whether the abuse directly causes the ADHD or whether the ADHD causes childhood abuse secondary to parents having to manage a child with difficult behaviors. In the homeless population people will often self-medicate with stimulants to help them focus—typically clients will tell you that stimulants will help them feel better but other people around them who they are using with are getting high.

Learning Disorders and Intellectual Disabilities Learning disorders are defined in DSM V as "Specific Learning Disorders" or in ICD 11 as "Developmental Learning Disorders" which can manifest in difficulties in reading, writing or mathematics. Learning disorders in intelligent children are often not diagnosed because they can perform at an average level but cause significant frustration and behavioral issues in school. Working in street medicine it is common to see people struggle with filling out forms or trying to navigate complex health or housing systems. Exact figures on the prevalence of difficulties in reading and writing in the homeless population are hard to come by but some estimates suggest at least 50% of people affected by homelessness have some difficulties with reading and writing [24]. A UK charity Literacy100 [25] exists to address the problems of literacy in the homeless. Clinically it is always helpful to directly ask people how well they can read and write. Learning how to read and write can be transformative for some and a qualitative study by Juchniewicz describes how literacy gives people a way to "rewrite" their lives and value their personal stories [26].

People with intellectual disabilities are common in the homeless population with systematic reviews estimating prevalences of 12–39% [27]. However intellectual disabilities are often missed so that again routine screening is often advised with the Learning Disability Screening Questionnaire (LDSQ) having high sensitivity (83%) and specificity (96%) in the homeless population when completed by staff [28]. The LDSQ has seven questions, three of the LDSQ items address skills related to understanding functions of a clock, reading and writing, two items address living independently or not, having employment or not, and two are about the experiences of receiving assistance at school or at home. The full LDSQ is available for purchase from GCM Records LLP [29].

7.3 The Effects of Cognitive Impairment

Cognitive impairment in homeless individuals significantly affects their ability to function and engage with support systems. Impaired memory and executive functioning can interfere with the ability to keep appointments, follow treatment plans, or navigate complex bureaucracies to access benefits and housing. People with cognitive impairment can present with challenging behaviors that cause them to not get treated in hospital or be barred from shelters. As a result, individuals with cognitive impairment are more likely to experience chronic homelessness and have repeated interactions with emergency services, the criminal justice system and hospitals [30].

Functional cognition refers to the ability to use cognitive abilities in everyday activities such as looking after themselves, working or socializing. This means that as well as identifying cognitive ability it is also important to assess how any cognitive impairment affect what people can do. One approach demonstrated in the literature on assessing brain injury in the homeless [31] is to use the World Health Organization Disability Assessment Schedule 2.0 (WHODAS 2.0) to assess any disability [32]. A scoping review of functional cognition in 37 studies covering 4850 homeless people [33] found a consistent effect of cognitive deficits on activities of daily living. They also found that cognitive impairment was related to time spent being homeless and did not improve after obtaining housing. The authors concluded that screening and identifying cognitive deficits was important so that strengths could be identified and appropriate supports could be put in place to transition to housing and stay housed. Moreover, cognitive impairments can make individuals more vulnerable to exploitation, victimization, and abuse. They may be less able to assess risks or protect themselves in precarious living situations. The stigma associated with cognitive and mental impairments further isolates individuals, exacerbating feelings of hopelessness and despair. Without appropriate recognition and support, these individuals are at heightened risk of deteriorating physical and mental health, social disconnection, and early mortality. Cognitive impairment can create a vicious cycle, where homelessness exacerbates cognitive decline, which in turn entrenches homelessness [1].

7.4 Assessing Capacity

An important consequence of cognitive impairment is on capacity to make decisions. This can affect a person's eligibility and need for services as well ability to care for their health problems. Generally capacity assessment is specific to a particular area such as capacity to consent to medical treatment and focuses on four questions—can the person consistently express a choice, do they understand the relevant information, can they understand the consequences of making a decision and can they apply that to their own circumstances [34].

In people who are homeless assessing capacity for decision-making is difficult because of potential effects from substance use and the environments where most testing takes place. When we are in the early days of establishing rapport with people, particularly people with obvious signs of psychosis and paranoia, it can be tricky. You meet someone who is profoundly ill but very wary of associating with anyone from the medical establishment. You may be more prone to introduce yourself simply as a nurse or a doctor than as a mental health clinician. This is a tricky line-sometimes trying to help people with their physical health stuff first (again returning to the idea of attending a wound or helping soak someone's feet!) feels much less daunting to people than opening up the vulnerabilities around mood, thoughts and anxieties. Attending to people's obvious health needs helps form a therapeutic alliance and sometimes this helps people start to divulge other areas of their life where they are needing help.

When it is very clear to the patients that they are seeing a mental health clinician it's good to be very clear about the boundaries. How much time do you have for the patient, how often can you see them? What organization do you work for? Being mindful that certain medications carry more stigma than others is important. Things like lithium and antipsychotics are medications that people can have profound negative associations with. In the Ottawa context, Seroquel (generic name is quetiapine) is known as "bug juice" for example, and is widely used in our local jail to help the inmates sleep. As a result, it has some street value as a sleep aide and some people really like it for that reason and some people really don't.

People may be unwilling to talk with you about antipsychotics, but they are willing to talk with you about medications for sleep for instance. The language that we use is important. If we recognize that someone may be psychotic and has little insight but wants something for sleep, offering antipsychotics for sleep and informing them of the potential risks/benefits of the medication without naming the class of drug seems beneficial to the patient.

Keep in mind that relationship is the key to everything we do. Informed consent is an ongoing process that needs to occur in this relationship. As we get to know each other, we provide the patient with information about their health status, diagnosis, treatment options, and prognosis. We get to know our patient's values and what is important to them, and this helps drive our conversations with our patients about their care. The patient should participate in the development and decision-making of the plan of care, including the right to consent to or refuse treatment [35]. One of the tools that is helpful sometimes when having difficult conversations with patients about their care is the wish-worry-wonder tool that comes from palliative care [36]. "I wish" allows for aligning with the patient's desires; "I worry" allows for expressing of your concerns in a sensitive manner; while "I wonder" allows you to subtly make a recommendation. For example, when suggesting starting medication to someone who is ambivalent about starting medication, this tool might be used something like this, "I wish that you didn't need to take medication. I worry that if you don't start medication that you are going to continue to suffer with these horrible thoughts and feelings about yourself. I wonder if you tried the medication for a month if we could come back together and see how you feel then."

When starting to work with people who are actively using substances daily, you may be under the assumption that people using substances don't have the capacity to make thoughtful decisions for themselves and their well-being. People who are actively using substances are not automatically incapable of making decisions for themselves and this is particularly important to be thoughtful about when people are actively using substances daily to survive and cope. However, it is important to be thoughtful about consent and capacity if someone is highly inebriated and putting themselves or others at risk. One of the times that a team can really be challenged ethically is when someone's substance use is putting their health at high risk. It's challenging when someone is in the throes of addiction to know if they are capable or not at times because the substance drives so much of their behavior. This is often as a team where I would suggest clinicians go in pairs to talk with the patient to see if they are getting the same perspective or feeling from the patient. There's been times with certain patients that the ethical dilemmas have been so challenging for our team that we have had the hospital ethicist come in on our medical rounds so that we can make sure we have offered every perspective and looked at all the options and know that as a team we did the best we could with a bad situation. Doing repeated assessments over time, involving others in the assessment for collaborative information and discussion about the process are ways to mitigate some of these difficulties.

There have been attempts to create questionnaires which are specific for the homeless population such as the Capacity Assessment Instrument for People who Misuse Substances (CAIP) which consists of 11 questions that are rated on a scale of 1 to 4 with higher scores indicating higher capacity [37]. Other standardized questionnaires for more general use include the Aid to Capacity Evaluation (ACE) [38] or the MacArthur Competence Assessment Tool-Treatment (MacCAT-T) [39] which both focus on decisions about medical treatment.

7.5 Assessment of Cognitive Impairment

Cognitive assessment in chaotic environments presents significant challenges; however, it is important to not forget the basics of history taking, mental state examination, and physical examination. A comprehensive approach should include:

History taking Gather information about current cognitive issues - Inquire about past cognitive problems and their progression - Assess the patient's ability to engage in conversation and answer simple questions.

A focused traumatic brain injury assessment A scoping review [40] recommended the Ohio State University Traumatic Brain Injury—Identification Method (OSU TBI-ID) [41] to screen for traumatic brain injury in people who are homeless. The OSU TBI-ID is not copyrighted and is a structured interview for eliciting a person's lifetime history of TBI that takes 3–5 minutes. There are five questions with supplementary questions.

(i) *In your lifetime, have you ever been hospitalized or treated in an emergency room following an injury to your head or neck? Think about any childhood injuries you remember or were told about.*

(ii) *In your lifetime, have you ever injured your head or neck in a car accident or from crashing some other moving vehicle like a bicycle, motorcycle or ATV?*
(iii) *In your lifetime, have you ever injured your head or neck in a fall or from being hit by something (for example, falling from a bike or horse, rollerblading, falling on ice, being hit by a rock)? Have you ever injured your head or neck playing sports or on the playground?*
(iv) *In your lifetime, have you ever injured your head or neck in a fight, from being hit by someone, or from being shaken violently? Have you ever been shot in the head?*
(v) *In your lifetime, have you ever been nearby when an explosion or a blast occurred? If you served in the military, think about any combat or training related incidents.*

If the answer is yes to any of these questions, ask: *Were you knocked out or did you lose consciousness (LOC)? If yes, how long? If no, were you dazed or did you have a gap in your memory from the injury? How old were you?*

A supplementary question is: *Have you ever lost consciousness from a drug overdose or being choked?*

Document the number and timing of head injuries—Determine the severity of injuries based on hospital admissions, duration of stay, and duration of memory loss—Evaluate any history of seizures, strokes, brain disorders (Parkinson's or Huntington's for example), brain infections such as meningitis, or prolonged exposure to heavy metals or pesticides.

Developmental history Ask about maternal health during pregnancy, including alcohol or drug use—Inquire about premature birth or postnatal hospitalization—Assess early childhood development milestones (Of course people who have experienced trauma early in life may have difficulty remembering details of their childhood).

Educational background Determine if special education or additional support was required—Identify any attention-related issues in the classroom setting—Note any history of stimulant or other medication use during childhood.

Brief physical examination Observe for tremors or involuntary movements—Check for head scars or other signs of previous injury—Assess overall physical appearance, noting any characteristics suggestive of specific conditions (for example fetal alcohol syndrome features)—Evaluate the patient's size relative to age, which may indicate a history of prematurity—Assess gross motor skills and gait—Evaluate speech patterns and articulation.

Sensory assessment Check visual acuity and hearing capabilities—Note any sensory sensitivities or deficits—If available an eye chart without letters (such as the Allen pictures chart or Tumbling E chart) can be used and some teams use a portable auto-refractor that can produce a prescription on the spot.

Behavioral observations Monitor the patient's attention span and concentration during the assessment—If you think that there is a disorder of attention, which is the defining feature of delirium, ask the person to name the months of the year backwards starting at December and ending in January (or if they can't do this try the days of the week backward from Sunday)—Observe social interaction skills and emotional regulation.

Cognitive screening tools Use brief, validated cognitive screening instruments suitable for chaotic settings—Focus on key domains such as orientation, memory, and executive function—Examples include the Montreal Cognitive Assessment (MoCA) [42] and the Mini-Mental State Examination (MMSE) [43], although these should be interpreted cautiously. Relying just on a numeric score can be misleading as deficits may be spread between the different domains or be restricted to just one area. Also, the MMSE is poor at detecting executive deficits as it is more focused on assessing memory, attention and language.

A scoping review of screening tools for cognitive impairment and traumatic brain injury in people who are homeless recommended the Trail Making Tests A and B as viable tools for screening for cognitive impairment in the homeless population [40]. The trail making test A asks the client to connect 25 randomly placed numbered circles in ascending order from 1 to 25. Trail making test B connects 24 randomly placed circles in ascending order alternating between numbers and letters (1-A-2-B…). Scoring is the number of seconds required to complete each task. More than one error or taking over 78 seconds for Trail A or 273 seconds for Trail B is in the lowest tenth percentile and is "deficient". The mean for Trail A is 29 seconds and Trail B is 75 seconds. Consider completing the WHODAS to determine the level of disability.

Collateral information When possible, gather information from family members or caregivers to corroborate the patient's history and current functioning. Does the patient have a friend who accompanies them a lot of the time. One of the things we come across a lot is that some of our more frail clients can function because of their social network, they have a community that can help them access food or get to the pharmacy for example. There is a highly protective aspect to the street community that can help mitigate the consequences of poor cognition. However, we also see our cognitively impaired clients being exploited, for example, having their bank cards repeatedly stolen, misplacing large amounts of money, or have "friends" who come around only at cheque time.

7.6 Intervention and Support

Interventions for homeless individuals with cognitive impairment should be multidisciplinary and adapted to their specific needs. Occupational therapists have training and skills to support individuals after brain injury and should be considered as a part of any street medicine team. Occupational therapists have an established role in rehabilitation clinics where there are established evidence based methods to address cognitive impairment [44] and there is an emerging interest in transferring these skills to homeless settings [45]. Housing First models that provide stable, permanent housing without preconditions do not in themselves appear to improve cognition [46] but they do create a setting where focused interventions may take place.

Cognitive remediation therapies with a focus on SMART (Specific, Measurable, Achievable, Realistic, Time limited) goals and specific activities, while resource-intensive, may offer benefit, especially if integrated into broader psychosocial support. There is some evidence for the effectiveness of this approach in homeless youth, but engaging people can be challenging [47]. Simple steps such as providing pocket diaries to patients or having visible calendars and other aides to orientation where people gather can be helpful. Pill organizers can be helpful especially if the person can't be seen daily. Clinicians also need to provide simple explanations and instructions with small well-defined goals. This can be backed up with written instructions at an appropriate reading age or drawings.

References

1. Burra TA, Stergiopoulos V, Rourke SB. A systematic review of cognitive deficits in homeless adults: implications for service delivery. The Canadian Journal of Psychiatry [Internet] 2009 [cited 2025 Mar 23];54(2):123–33. Available from: https://journals.sagepub.com/doi/abs/10.1177/070674370905400210
2. Ennis N, Roy S, Topolovec-Vranic J. Memory impairment among people who are homeless: a systematic review. Memory [Internet] 2015 [cited 2025 Mar 23];23(5):695–713. Available from: https://www.tandfonline.com/doi/abs/10.1080/09658211.2014.921714
3. Depp CA, Vella L, Orff HJ, Twamley EW. A quantitative review of cognitive functioning in homeless adults. J Nervous Mental Dis [Internet]. 2015 [cited 2025 Mar 23];203(2):126–31. Available from: https://journals.lww.com/jonmd/fulltext/2015/02000/a_quantitative_review_of_cognitive_functioning_in.9.aspx
4. Stone B, Dowling S, Cameron A. Cognitive impairment and homelessness: a scoping review. Health Soc Care Community [Internet]. 2019 [cited 2025 Mar 23];27(4):e125–42. Available from: https://onlinelibrary-wiley-com.proxy.bib.uottawa.ca/doi/full/10.1111/hsc.12682
5. Backer TE, Howard EA. Cognitive impairments and the prevention of homelessness: research and practice review. J Prim Prev [Internet]. 2007 [cited 2025 Mar 30];28(3–4):375–88. Available from: https://pubmed.ncbi.nlm.nih.gov/17549638/
6. Stubbs JL, Thornton AE, Sevick JM, Silverberg ND, Barr AM, Honer WG, et al. Traumatic brain injury in homeless and marginally housed individuals: a systematic review and meta-analysis. Lancet Public Health. Elsevier Ltd. 2020;5:e19–32.
7. Bennett N, Chung JS, Lundstern MS, Bymaster A. Traumatic brain injury and its risk factors in a homeless population. Arch Phys Med Rehabil. 2024;105(12):2286–93.
8. Rigney G, Leith J, Lennon M, Reeves A, Chrisinger B. The Association of Traumatic Brain Injury with neurologic and psychiatric illnesses among individuals experiencing homelessness: a systematic review and meta-analysis. J Health Care Poor Underserved. 2022;33(2):685–701.
9. Gilchrist G, Morrison DS. Prevalence of alcohol related brain damage among homeless hostel dwellers in Glasgow. Eur J Public Health [Internet]. 2005;15(6):587–8. Available from: https://academic.oup.com/eurpub/article/15/6/587/440068
10. Winstanley EL, Mahoney JJ, Castillo F, Comer SD. Neurocognitive impairments and brain abnormalities resulting from opioid-related overdoses: a systematic review. Drug Alcohol Depend [Internet]. 2021 [cited 2025 Mar 23];226:108838. Available from: https://pmc.ncbi.nlm.nih.gov/articles/PMC8889511/
11. Potvin S, Pelletier J, Grot S, Hébert C, Barr A, Lecomte T. Cognitive deficits in individuals with methamphetamine use disorder: a meta-analysis. Addict Behav. 2018;(80):154–60.
12. Almeida PP, de Araujo Filho GM, Malta SM, Laranjeira RR, Marques ACRP, Bressan RA, et al. Attention and memory deficits in crack-cocaine users persist over four weeks of abstinence. J Subst Abus Treat. 2017;(81):73–8.

13. De Sousa T, Andrichik A, Prestera E, Rush K, Tano C, Wheeler M, et al. The 2023 Annual Homelessness Assessment Report (AHAR) to Congress Part 1: Point-In-Time Estimates of Homelessness December 2023 Acknowledgements Design and Production 2023.
14. Ross HM, Dzenga P, Myers M, Squires A, Duncan S, Caradine J, et al. Dementia and mild cognitive impairment screening in an emergency homeless shelter. Alzheimer's Dementia [Internet] 2024 [cited 2025 Mar 23];20(5):3666–70. Available from: https://onlinelibrary-wiley-com.proxy.bib.uottawa.ca/doi/full/10.1002/alz.13763
15. Booth RG, Dasgupta M, Forchuk C, Shariff SZ. Prevalence of dementia among people experiencing homelessness in Ontario, Canada: a population-based comparative analysis. Lancet Public Health. 2024;9(4):e240–9.
16. Menon J, Kantipudi SJ, Mani A, Radhakrishnan R. Cognitive functioning and functional ability in women with schizophrenia and homelessness. Schizophr Res Cogn. 2025;(39):100338.
17. Chudley AE, Conry J, Cook JL, Loock C, Rosales T, LeBlanc N. Fetal alcohol spectrum disorder: Canadian guidelines for diagnosis. CMAJ [Internet]. 2005 [cited 2025 Apr 1];172(5 suppl):S1–21. Available from: https://www.cmaj.ca/content/172/5_suppl/S1
18. Fazari G, Bibr C, Harding K. A place to call home: addressing housing needs for individuals with fetal alcohol spectrum disorder. 2024 [cited 2025 Apr 1]; Available from: https://canfasd.ca/wp-content/uploads/publications/Housing-Issue-Paper_Final.pdf
19. Churchard A, Ryder M, Greenhill A, Mandy W. The prevalence of autistic traits in a homeless population. Autism [Internet]. 2019 [cited 2025 Apr 6];23(3):665–76. Available from: https://doi.org/10.1177/1362361318768484.
20. Boilson AM, Churchard A, Connolly M, Casey B, Sweeney MR. Screening for Autism spectrum condition through inner city homeless services in the Republic of Ireland. 2023 [cited 2025 Apr 6];53:3987–98. Available from: https://doi.org/10.1007/s10803-022-05669-x
21. Stone B, Cameron A, Dowling S. The autistic experience of homelessness: Implications from a narrative enquiry. Autism [Internet]. 2023 [cited 2025 Apr 6];27(2):489–99. Available from: https://journals-sagepub-com.proxy.bib.uottawa.ca/doi/full/10.1177/13623613221105091
22. Denis C, Boucaud-Maitre D, Brunelin J, Jurek L, Vallet W, Demily C. Prevalence of attention deficit hyperactivity disorder in homeless children and adolescents: a systematic review and meta-analysis. Dialogues Clin Neurosci [Internet]. 2025 [cited 2025 Apr 9];27(1):86–97. Available from: https://www.tandfonline.com/doi/full/10.1080/19585969.2025.2486355
23. Bali P, Sonuga-Barke E, Mohr-Jensen C, Demontis D, Minnis H. Is there evidence of a causal link between childhood maltreatment and attention deficit/hyperactivity disorder? A systematic review of prospective longitudinal studies using the Bradford-Hill criteria. JCPP Adv [Internet]. 2023 [cited 2025 Apr 9];3(4). Available from: https://pubmed.ncbi.nlm.nih.gov/38054051/
24. Reading Counts: why English and maths skills matter in tackling homelessness | St Mungo's [Internet]. [cited 2025 Apr 13]. Available from: https://www.mungos.org/research-publication/reading-counts-why-english-and-maths-skills-matter-in-tackling-homelessness/
25. Home | Literacy100 [Internet]. [cited 2025 Apr 22]. Available from: https://www.literacy100.org/
26. Juchniewicz MM. Visible voices: literacy identity and the invisible homeless. J Adolesc Adult Lit. 2012;55(6):505–15.
27. Durbin A, Isaacs B, Mauer-Vakil D, Connelly J, Steer L, Roy S, et al. Intellectual disability and homelessness: a synthesis of the literature and discussion of how supportive housing can support wellness for people with intellectual disability. Curr Dev Disord Rep [Internet]. 2018 [cited 2025 Apr 9];5(3):125–31. Available from: https://link-springer-com.proxy.bib.uottawa.ca/article/10.1007/s40474-018-0141-6
28. McKenzie K, Murray G, Metcalfe D, Robson R, Kaczmar M, Shirley A. Using the learning disability screening questionnaire to help identify people with an intellectual disability in homeless services. J Appl Res Intellect Disabil [Internet]. 2023 [cited 2025 Apr 9];36(6):1319–25. Available from: https://onlinelibrary-wiley-com.proxy.bib.uottawa.ca/doi/full/10.1111/jar.13150

29. LDSQ | GCM RECORDS LLP [Internet]. [cited 2025 Apr 22]. Available from: https://gcmrecordsllp.co.uk/the-learning-disability-screening-questionnaire-ldsq/
30. To MJ, O'Brien K, Palepu A, Hubley AM, Farrell S, Aubry T, et al. Healthcare utilization, legal incidents, and victimization following traumatic brain injury in homeless and vulnerably housed individuals: a prospective cohort study. J Head Trauma Rehabil [Internet] 2015 [cited 2025 Apr 23];30(4):270–6. Available from: https://pubmed.ncbi.nlm.nih.gov/24651000/
31. Synovec CE, Berry S. Addressing brain injury in health care for the homeless settings: a pilot model for provider training. Work. 2020;65(2):285–96.
32. WHO Disability Assessment Schedule (WHODAS 2.0) [Internet]. [cited 2025 Apr 21]. Available from: https://www.who.int/standards/classifications/international-classification-of-functioning-disability-and-health/who-disability-assessment-schedule
33. Synovec CE, Leonie Boland B, Westover L, Author C, Synovec C. Evaluation of functional cognition in people experiencing homelessness: a scoping review. Int J Homelessness [Internet]. 2023 [cited 2025 Apr 23];3(3):302–38. Available from: https://ojs.lib.uwo.ca/index.php/ijoh/article/view/16454
34. Appelbaum PS. Clinical practice. Assessment of patients' competence to consent to treatment. N Engl J Med [Internet]. 2007 [cited 2025 Apr 22];357(18):1834–40. Available from: https://pubmed.ncbi.nlm.nih.gov/17978292/
35. Farmer L, Lundy A. Informed consent: ethical and legal considerations for advanced practice nurses. J Nurse Pract. 2017;13(2):124–30.
36. CAPC program. Communication Support Frameworks.
37. Taylor D. CAIPS Capacity Assessment Instrument for People who Misuse Substances [Internet]. 2014 [cited 2025 Apr 22]. Available from: https://smartsexresource.com/wp-content/uploads/resources/CAIPS-prototype-8-Jan-2015.pdf?x85715
38. Etchells E. Aid To Capacity Evaluation (ACE). Can Med Assoc J [Internet]. 1996 [cited 2025 Apr 22];155:657–61. Available from: www.jcb.utoronto.ca/tools/ace.shtml1
39. Grisso T, Appelbaum PS, Hill-Fotouhi C. The MacCAT-T: a clinical tool to assess patients' capacities to make treatment decisions. Psychiatr Serv [Internet]. 1997 [cited 2025 Apr 22];48(11):1415–9. Available from: https://pubmed.ncbi.nlm.nih.gov/9355168/
40. Fearn-Smith EM, Scanlan JN, Hancock N. Exploring and mapping screening tools for cognitive impairment and traumatic brain injury in the homelessness context: a scoping review. Int J Environ Res Public Health [Internet] 2023 [cited 2025 Mar 23];20(4):3440. Available from: https://www.mdpi.com/1660-4601/20/4/3440/htm
41. Corrigan JD, Bogner J. Ohio State University traumatic brain injury identification method. Encyclopedia of clinical neuropsychology [Internet] 2018 [cited 2025 Apr 6];2502–4. Available from: https://link.springer.com/referenceworkentry/10.1007/978-3-319-57111-9_9053
42. Nasreddine ZS, Phillips NA, Bédirian V, Charbonneau S, Whitehead V, Collin I, et al. The Montreal Cognitive Assessment, MoCA: a brief screening tool for mild cognitive impairment. J Am Geriatr Soc [Internet]. 2005 [cited 2025 Apr 6];53(4):695–9. Available from: https://pubmed.ncbi.nlm.nih.gov/15817019/
43. Folstein MF, Folstein SE, McHugh PR. "Mini-mental state". A practical method for grading the cognitive state of patients for the clinician. J Psychiatr Res [Internet]. 1975 [cited 2025 Apr 6];12(3):189–98. Available from: https://pubmed.ncbi.nlm.nih.gov/1202204/
44. Cicerone KD, Dams-O'Connor K, Eberle R, Fraas M, Ganci K, Langenbahn D, et al. The ACRM cognitive rehabilitation manual & textbook: translating evidence-based recommendations into practice [Internet]. 2nd ed. ACRM Publishing; 2022 [cited 2025 Apr 26]. 463 p. Available from: https://books.google.com/books/about/ACRM_Cognitive_Rehabilitation_Manual_Tex.html?id=Z0fqzgEACAAJ
45. Synovec C. Occupational therapy's role in addressing the needs of people experiencing homelessness [Internet]. 2022 [cited 2025 Apr 26]. Available from: https://www.occupationaltherapy.com/articles/occupational-therapy-s-role-in-5494-5494

46. Stergiopoulos V, Naidu A, Schuler A, Bekele T, Nisenbaum R, Jbilou J, et al. Housing stability and neurocognitive functioning in homeless adults with mental illness: a subgroup analysis of the At Home/Chez Soi Study. Front Psychiatry [Internet]. 2019 [cited 2025 Apr 23];10. Available from: https://pubmed.ncbi.nlm.nih.gov/31849725/
47. Medalia A, Saperstein AM, Huang Y, Lee S, Ronan EJ. Cognitive skills training for homeless transition-age youth: feasibility and pilot efficacy of a community based randomized controlled trial. J Nerv Ment Dis [Internet]. 2017 [cited 2025 Apr 23];205(11):859–66. Available from: https://pubmed.ncbi.nlm.nih.gov/28937497/

8 Chaos

A middle-aged white male, "John" with a large white beard and a bright twinkle in his blue eyes who was new to our managed alcohol supportive housing facility and getting accustomed to living with people again described how he felt like there were two people living inside of him—his "drunk self" and his "sober self." Keep in mind that his "sober self" was still using but in a managed way where he wasn't intoxicated. When he talked about his drunk self, he talked about wanting to be alone, about not being able to trust himself around others, about his chaos, about his feelings of wanting to die, about his deep-rooted feelings of unworthiness, about seeing bugs and hearing voices and about passing out drunk in places he didn't know. He was deeply troubled by this part of himself and didn't know what drove him to this place—he talked about it in all sorts of ugly, dark terms. This was a man who had grown up in a large family of drinkers, who had been encouraged to start drinking alcohol as a child by his parents. However, during his adulthood he had periods of stability and decreased drinking while he had his kids and family and was running a farm. When he talked about his sober self, he spoke about enjoying the company of others, of enjoying being taken care of, of showering and paying attention to his health and hygiene and of wanting to reconnect with his family.

Over time I got to know John and we shared a lot of laughs together. He was a big man with a big belly and a matching laugh and could be quite intimidating when he was drunk. We connected well, maybe because we both shared histories of growing up on a farm or because I laughed at all his jokes. I shared hope with him, telling him that I had met other patients in similar situations before, and that with some medication, with some time, with him making the effort to drink only the alcohol provided by the program, with him connecting with others and finding his place in his housing that I saw him returning to stability and a sense of "normalcy." He tried some mood stabilizers to help with his labile moods and impulse control issues and found them useful. We developed care plans for the staff of how to engage with him when he drank outside and returned to the program intoxicated and verbally abusive towards the staff.

S. Hatcher et al., *Street Mental Health Handbook*,
https://doi.org/10.1007/978-3-032-00663-9_8

This isn't an isolated conversation as mental health clinicians working with patients with profound substance use and mental health issues. This is something we hear from people quite regularly, of this sense of multiple selves, of this lack of understanding of the chaos and trauma that drives our patients into dark places. Of this profound sense of disconnectedness from the self. As street clinicians, part of our role is managing our patients' chaos and helping them understand these parts of themselves. Often when first encountering people the list of needs they have can be quite overwhelming and we ourselves can become exhausted. Are we only there with a patient to do an assessment, provide a diagnosis, and help connect people with treatment? Or are we also helping people access food, shelter, clothing, and basic needs? We can get caught up in the struggle of what our role is, what we are there to do. Being prepared by having lists of local resources, carrying some basic needs with you, and a sense of what you should/shouldn't help with may be helpful in managing this chaos, both for you and the patient.

The chaos really speaks to the importance of working in teams, to have other people we can refer to and talk things through with. I carry a notebook and write down what the patient's concerns were, what needs followed up on, certain statements that were made that I want to get down in my clinical notes, which all helps me with my charting later in the day and to remember what I need to follow up on. When I'm with a paranoid person, I keep my notebook tucked away and quickly scribble my notes down after or text myself. Carrying the notebook can get in the way of being my authentic self and being fully present with people in the "human" way of getting down to their level, making eye contact with them, seeing the expressions that pass on their faces as they say certain things, or look like I'm being too official, or "writing someone up."

8.1 Helping Frontline Staff Manage the Chaos

Part of the work of helping to manage the patients' chaos, is also to help manage the staff's chaos. For staff who have never worked with someone like John before, it's hard for them to imagine him getting better, imagine his behaviors changing and to not become intimidated by him. Part of our work as street clinicians is to educate shelter staff, drop-in program staff, outreach staff etc. about what is reasonable to expect of patients, how to approach patients in consistent, empathetic ways, and how to deescalate patients for example. We teach the staff that our patients' behavior isn't going to change overnight, but with time, empathy and connection, and consistent responding to behaviors, we would expect to see a reduction in behaviors such as aggression.

Working with frontline staff around these types of behaviors takes a lot of work and effort and a lot of role modeling of how to respond to behaviors. At times I have developed scripts for how staff can respond to patients. For example, we've had patients with profound brain injuries that become aggressive whenever they are told "no." The intervention was teaching the staff how to say no in a different way without using that word. For example, if the patient approached the desk asking for a sandwich and there were no meals available it was "I will be happy to get you a sandwich in an hour when they are available." At first sometimes the staff are resistant with scripts, or think you are being "soft." You need the staff to buy in if your intervention is going to work. You have to role model these interventions and have the staff see your calm, kind and firm presentation, the way that you follow up with the patient to make sure they are fed when the sandwich is available, etc. Teach staff how by engaging in kind, consistent ways that they will get patients more engaged in their care and more willing to follow direction.

Frontline staff in places like shelters are working with patients 24/7 and therefore deal with much more unpleasant aspects of the work than we do as clinicians who often are only in these places for small chunks of time. Frontline workers have far less training, are often black staff that encounter significant racist behavior from patients and are being paid far less and often living close to the poverty line themselves. Part of our work may be helping to coach frontline staff on managing their own internal chaos and compassion fatigue. How can we expect staff to engage in trauma-informed ways with patients if they are not being treated well themselves? This is the tricky balancing act of this work at times, the oppression our patients face and the oppression the staff working frontline jobs can face. Coauthor Simon Hatcher says to me often "who is the patient we are taking care of in this situation Kim?". So often our work as clinicians doing street work is about navigating staff concerns about patients. Be thoughtful about what intervention you are providing and who is it for. Sometimes interventions for staff (i.e. education) are a good use of your time and a way to help provide better care for a larger number of patients. Sometimes one staff member can be very vocal about their distress, but it may not be reflective of the rest of the team's distress or the patient's distress. It takes skill and time to be able to discern these things.

8.2 Helping Ourselves and Our Staff Manage the Chaos

From a staff wellness perspective, the chaos can be quite challenging and is part of why this environment isn't suited to everyone or sometimes doesn't work for staff at certain points in their lives (i.e. if your personal life is also feeling quite chaotic). Part of the joy of street psychiatry can be the adrenalin of not being in the same place every day, of not knowing what the day will bring, of getting to walk around your city and explore places you might not otherwise go. For some street clinicians who prefer to have a sense of control over our days and time this can get overwhelming. The day gets away from us very quickly when you go to an encampment expecting to meet one or two patients and instead find many patients interested in talking with you. Sometimes my most uncomfortable moments happen when I am talking with a patient I was expecting to meet up with and then they have a friend who is also desperately trying to engage with me at the same time. How do we prioritize who needs to get seen that day or how much time we can spend with one patient, particularly if it takes us an extraordinary amount of time just to find them? This is something important to be mindful of when interviewing staff or thinking about who makes up your team. If you are a street psychiatry team that is just starting out, you need clinicians who are creative, who are happy to work in the "gray," and who are very flexible. As your work in the field continues, your organization gets bigger, you will find that your team needs more policies and procedures, and less "gray" and the tricky balancing act becomes between keeping your nimbleness to be "for the people" and being able to run an organization.

Part of the challenge of working in the chaos is knowing and maintaining our boundaries. This is a struggle especially for those of us who get into the work with big ambitions of saving the world or become fixated with our patient's traumatic story. It's hard to say no to patients or not to be able to do all the things we want to do for people when our patients live in such dire circumstances. However, so many people on the streets have had well-meaning people make promises that they didn't keep, they find it hard to trust us. The need to be realistic with what we are not able to do and what we don't have control over is more about carefully tending to the relationship with someone sleeping rough and checking our own ambitions at the door. The therapeutic relationship is such a small tender thing that it needs to be held gently. In our passion for helping, our overcommitting and failing can break the thing we must nurture the most. Is this our own failing or are there bigger systemic gaps that we are trying to fill by running ourselves ragged? Knowing the balance of when we need to go above and beyond because it's the right thing to do and when we need to say no is hard and often takes us talking with coworkers, our supervisor, a therapist to manage. This is the part when we also need to practice self-compassion, would we expect others to do what we are expecting of ourselves?

8.3 Lived Experience of the Chaos

Tabitha Morris, one of Ottawa Inner City Health's beloved peer workers and now a peer manager, has brought so much wisdom and radical love to our team and the work that we do. During COVID she worked as a peer worker in our COVID isolation unit for the homeless, helping provide harm reduction services to our clients so they didn't have to make the choice between being able to continue to access their drugs and receive medical care. Tabitha also worked with community partners to create quarterly community funerals to honour community members we had lost during that quarter. She collected photographs and each person that is memorialized has a special funeral card made for them describing who they were and what people miss about them. Currently Tabitha is helping our organization implement the Life Process Program by Dr. Stanton Peele. She is collaborating with peer case managers in each of our supportive housing programs and our safe injection site to engage with clients around their values, motivation, life skills, community and relationships.

When I do outreach with Tabitha it's so much easier to approach the street entrenched clients. Tabitha is this warm, smiley woman giving out hugs to everyone and laughing and sharing a smoke. She has the trust of both men and women alike, so when I get the pleasure of walking around with her, I have this easier "in" with people. She introduces me as an old friend and has me cleaning wounds, listening to lungs, talking with someone about their recent sexual assault, or trying to help get someone on treatment for their psychosis. It always makes me feel better because even if I can't follow up with someone or find them again to follow up, I know there is a good chance Tabitha will. All her years of street living and now peer work mean she has a lot of good clinical skills; her knowledge and her relationships are an expertise I won't ever have. We have fun going out together and I think we both always feel good at the end of a day together, surprised by how much we can accomplish together.

Tabitha has taught our organization so much about the importance of building community and really is our expert in community development. The following is her words about the chaos of street life.

> If you ask someone what they most need while they are at the shelter or sleeping rough on the street, they will say "housing". "All I need is housing and everything else will get better". What is hard is to watch is that once someone gets housed, they often end up back at our services, back on the street, back with their COMMUNITY. While folks are on the street or in shelters – a community feel develops. Once housed, folks feel isolated, lonely, alone and bored. Often home is an empty apartment with no connection to the outside world.
>
> Housing workers tell their newly housed clients not to have guests, or to tell folks where they live in fear they will likely lose their housing or experience a home takeover. For many of the people with overwhelming substance use and mental health, there is a big chance they may lose their housing and return to the street or shelter. Reasons vary but include being unclean, damage to the apartment, long-staying visitors, traffic, noise, or, more often than not, a rent subsidy that wasn't renewed.
>
> Community needs to be created, norms need to be taught and modeled. Housing is a part of the answer but there is so much more that needs to go into this. We need to invest in sustainably diverse communities that have services for all, that are welcoming for all – communities of humans. Let's bring back "IT TAKES A VILLAGE."

8.4 The Hard Work of Being Homeless

The hard work of being homeless refers to the constant effort and struggle individuals experiencing homelessness must put in to find a place to sleep each night, secure meals, protect belongings, navigate public systems to access resources, and deal with the psychological stress of instability, all while often facing social stigma and limited access to support services.

Key aspects of the "hard work" of being homeless include:

Finding shelter: Constantly searching for a safe place to sleep, whether in shelters, public spaces, or temporary accommodations, which can involve navigating rules, waiting lists, and conflicts with other people. On the streets or in shelters there is no sense of privacy or having personal space. People describe sleeping regularly with rats or bugs on them. Brett Feldman, *Director of Street Medicine at the Keck School of Medicine of USC* and the Vice Chair of the Street Medicine Institute, notes that streets sweeps in the guise of cleaning up a space for the purpose of public health really tells people sleeping rough that they are garbage too. The impact of constantly being treated not only as unwanted, but as trash, on a person's soul causes what he calls a spiritual poverty.

Accessing necessities: Securing food through food banks, meal programs, or scavenging, managing limited access to clean water and sanitation facilities.

Protecting belongings: Always carrying all personal items with them, needing to be vigilant against theft, and finding ways to keep belongings clean and dry.

Navigating bureaucracy: Dealing with complex application processes for government assistance, housing programs, and other services, often requiring extensive documentation and repeated visits to different agencies. The need for an address, an ID, birth certificate, clean clothing when applying for jobs/services.

Managing mental health: Coping with the psychological stress of uncertainty, social isolation, and the constant struggle to meet basic needs, which can exacerbate existing mental health issues.

Maintaining personal hygiene: Finding ways to shower and clean themselves when access to facilities and clothing is limited.

Dealing with social stigma: Facing prejudice and discrimination from others due to their homeless status, impacting self-esteem and access to opportunities. Being denied access to basic services like bathrooms or a place to sit down. Racial discrimination.

Weather challenges: Enduring extreme weather conditions without adequate shelter, posing significant risks to health and safety.

Transportation: Not being able to get places where they live as there is no transit in those areas or they can't afford transit. Our patients often walk excessively long distances and as a result their feet can suffer significant health consequences.

Time: Not knowing the time or date, everything is based on surviving the present moment. The sense of what the future brings is overwhelming and can fill people with dread because there is a sense of death looming [4, 5, 16, 21, 22].

Being homeless is hard work. It is confusing being told different information by people who are "supposed to" be helping. Having to walk to different locations to be able to eat, to access a shower, to access clothing, to meet with your health care provider, all while carrying all the stuff you own on you so it doesn't get stolen or lost. Never getting to have a shower with hot water or have privacy in the shower. Having to sleep with multiple other strangers in the same room or outside with bugs and rats crawling and biting at you. Constantly sleeping with one eye open, becoming a hypervigilant person so that your stuff doesn't get stolen, so you don't get raped, in case the police come to break up your tent. Wanting desperately to get out of this life, to connect with the case manager about housing, and welfare, and your lost ID. But the case manager is never in their office and half the time you don't know what time it is or what day of the week it is. You haven't had a good sleep in days, you're irritable, you're hungry, you're dirty. You're starting to believe that maybe you deserve all of this. Everyone around you is high, or mentally ill and if they aren't they are leaving the shelter…going to the mall, going to the library, going somewhere where they can blend in and escape this craziness for a bit. You are looking for something to give you energy, to help you sleep, to help you not feel so lonely and overwhelmed with the shame of living this life.

Part of the hard work of being homeless is maintaining one's mental well-being and not being triggered of past trauma in the violence and chaos of the street environment. For our Indigenous clients, being homeless can be a return to living in a space that reminds them of trauma. Some of our clients who have been in residential schools have told us that the line-up of beds in the shelters reminded them of their time in residential schools. Our Indigenous clients talk about how difficult it is to be cared for by staff that don't speak their language or look like them or have any familiarity with their land or culture. A lot of the institutional practices that happen in shelters like having to ask for your belongings reinforces colonial trauma and contributes to Indigenous clients feeling highly triggered and hypervigilant in shelter surroundings. Many Indigenous clients talk about the need to do care differently because of their experiences of colonization and of facing racism in mainstream health care settings. Unfortunately, during my time as a street nurse, I have experienced several Indigenous women that I have been working with go missing or be murdered near the shelter and witnessed the lack of police engagement around the safety needs of Indigenous women. This has been heartbreaking to bear witness to and at times has pushed us to despair. As an organization we have put significant efforts into building trust with our Indigenous clients, including funding Indigenous healers for our clients to meet with and providing Truth and Reconciliation Training to all our staff.

For clients who identify as trans, there are significant safety concerns. If they stay in shelters or are even allowed in shelters, there is often discourse about which gender do they sleep with, what bathrooms are they are allowed to use. They are at extreme risk for violence. For trans-women and cis-women it is difficult to have your period while on the street and to be able to access bathrooms and sanitary napkins. Some women talk about the safety of wearing multiple layers, of being less attractive. Females experience profound levels of sexual violence on the streets. Sometimes the safest thing for a female is being in a violent relationship because her partner, although abusive, keeps her safe from everyone else and she is only being abused by one abuser. Trying to do safety planning with patients who are experiencing intimate partner violence on the streets is particularly complex, especially for patients who are using substances or have histories of violence and who have very limited choices as far as where they can stay.

Canadian and American cities are becoming more and more diverse and as a result we see the homeless population becoming more diverse as well. It is hard work being homeless and navigating a new country when you don't speak the language, and no one knows how to engage with you in a culturally appropriate way. Unfortunately, we now see people on the streets who are brand new to Canada. Shelters and our street health teams are woefully underprepared to meet the needs of these clients. We are meeting more and more people coming from other countries with significant complex comorbid health issues and very different experiences of engaging with health care and cultural understandings of health. There are significant language barriers and identification issues that make it very hard to help these patients, never mind the profound sense of isolation and trauma that many of these patients' experience.

8.5 Thinking About Time: Clock Time Versus Street Time

Our patients are prioritizing survival daily. They spend their time moving between community organizations to access their basic needs. We hear our patients talk about their desires for structure, routine, consistency and organization in their lives, and struggling to maintain their health and wellness and sobriety without it [13]. Future planning is of limited use because so much of life is out of one's personal control. The level of sensory stimulation is quite high. People often don't have access to a clock or calendar and can become disoriented because of this. Countless times patients have asked me for the time of day and been shocked by the answer, thinking it was 12 h ahead of what it was. For our patients that use substances and go on long "drug trips," they sometimes go days without sleeping and then sleep for days and are not aware of the passing of time. It never fails to surprise me as someone who is always planning my next meal in my head that when I talk with people that our patients can't remember the last time they ate or the last time they slept. No wonder they are agitated or lose their cool with staff when they told them lunch wasn't for another couple of hours!

What does this mean for us as clinicians working with this population? It means our patients aren't really functioning by the same clock we are. Trying to set up appointments with patients can sometimes be productive but requires a level of functioning that people who are on survival mode just don't have. How are we designing our services to see patients when they are most available? If we are thinking of people being in survival mode, sometimes the very best time to catch people is to meet them at places where they must go. For example, sometimes I will leave notes for people at the pharmacy if I want to communicate appointments or other important messages to them. Consider using the Housed Beds tool that Corinne Feldman, Brett Feldman and Joel Hunt developed for taking the history of an unsheltered person that includes things like where the person spends their time in order to be able to find them when needed or if their encampment gets swept. https://bettercareplaybook.org/resources/housed-beds-clinical-tool-taking-history-unsheltered-homeless-patient.

So often when I am first encountering people and trying to engage and they are in survival mode, I find myself getting to know them by helping them out with necessities like accessing clothing. It's a very different way of working with someone than you would find in a traditional clinic model where patients come to you because they have a clear problem they want you to help them fix and you often have the skillset to fix it. Sometimes our patients come to us clearly wanting help with their mental health issue, but so often staff or friends or community members are referring patients who usually have no insight into how ill they are presenting. The number of times I've worked with someone who is highly paranoid for months, walking by and saying hello to eventually have them respond back to me and let me give them a foot bath and rub their feet with lotion and feed them and talk to me …this is the story of my life as a street nurse. Simon still shakes his head in confusion at me after I've introduced someone to him and the patient has talked with him for 5 min and I am so excited by this. Time is a dubious thing when you're on survival mode and when you're trying to engage someone for their life.

8.6 Involuntary Commitment and Competing Priorities

We are in a complex time when it comes to thinking about our patient's legal rights and their autonomy. A lot of negative media and political attention has recently been focused on the growing rates of homelessness, encampments and how to respond to the crisis of overdose deaths. There have been growing calls to consider forced substance use treatment and involuntary commitment.

For example, in 2022 in California legislators approved the Community Assistance, Recovery and Empowerment Act which allows family members and first responders to ask judges to issue treatment plans including involuntary psychiatric holds. Advocates for this have argued that not helping people who are seriously ill and living in horrible conditions on the street is inhumane. The shift is dividing people who care for people with mental illness and/or substance use disorders over the very meaning of compassion and which rights should take precedence: civil rights like freedom of movement and medical consent? Or the right to appropriate medical care in a crisis? [2]. This is a tricky issue for us as street mental health clinicians who care for patients who have repeatedly been failed by different systems. As street clinicians we have a strong sense of going to our patients, of meeting them where they are at, of providing care based on our patient's autonomy and of needing to do care differently not only to meet our patient's needs but also to respond to the trauma of the different care systems that have gone before us and damaged our patient's belief in being able to receive safe care.

Involuntary commitment is a kind of force used in health care, that does limit the liberty of a person whose agency and options are already restricted by homelessness. It does have the potential to cause your patient to distrust the health care system. Are you committing someone because they are making bad decisions and are fully aware of the potential outcomes or because they genuinely don't have the capacity to realize the outcomes of their decisions? We are ethically obligated not only to minimize the trauma of using force but also to respond to patients with compassion and regard for their dignity to preserve the therapeutic capacity of the patient-clinician relationship [19]. Sometimes our decision to form or not form someone is based on the systems' level of overwhelm. If we know that there are no beds available on the mental health units in the local hospital we may do our very best to not form someone and possibly erode the therapeutic relationship when there is a very low probability of that person being given the care we are looking at for them to receive in hospital.

We encounter people in horrible living situations where we are watching people slowly deteriorate to the point where they are at risk of losing a limb or being in a grave medical state because of lack of competence to care for themselves, but the hospitals simply won't keep our patients because they are using substances and think they are "choosing" this lifestyle. On one hand when people are incapable, we would like to see the system step in more and help protect people. We have experienced our clients after we have involuntarily committed them asking us why we didn't do it sooner. We are distressed by the ethical dilemma of the situation; both not wanting the negative aspects of paternalism (coercion) but wanting the positive aspects of it (taking care of someone who is unable to do it themselves). It's tough to reconcile these two things because we can cause harm whether we engage in paternalism or not.

On the other hand, if people are capable of making their own decisions, even if these decisions are not necessarily in their best interest, people should be able to maintain their autonomy. We do not want to see a return to re-institutionalization, especially when the community supports that were necessary to support de-institutionalization were never put into place. Like many areas around the world, California is also facing a shortage of psychiatric facilities, voluntary treatment facilities, the health care staff needed to operate these facilities and housing with the appropriate supports. Advocates for the homeless and marginalized people express particular concern that racialized minorities who are overrepresented in the homeless population and overdiagnosed with schizophrenia, will now be disproportionately targeted for forced hospitalization and treatment. As well, there is very little evidence that forced treatment for substance use is effective, and many concerns that this would be harmful for people and trauma-reinforcing. For example, coauthor Liz Frye had a Black patient who had tried to kill himself the night before she saw him and she ultimately decided not to hospitalize him (even though she thought there was still a high risk of suicide) because locking him up in a hospital would've made him more at risk because of how severe his PTSD from prison was.There are significant concerns about the risk for death from overdose after compulsory treatment. For example, in Massachusetts, people who were involuntarily committed for drug treatment were twice as likely to die from an overdose as those who received treatment willingly [6].

At a time when voluntary mental health and substance use treatments are so inaccessible to our patients, it's tough to justify violating people's rights to engage them in involuntary treatments [3]. Because we are often working with some of the most ill and complex patients, there are absolutely times when we have no other choice but to petition for someone to be held against their will. At these times it is important that we use our voice to advocate for people. Take the time to connect with the team at the admitting hospital. Write letters outlining the interventions your team has tried with the patient, how long it took your team to engage in relationship/rapport with that patient, their living conditions, their deteriorating health, the behaviors they exhibit with others, etc. Clinicians at the hospital don't understand the context of the street and are not as familiar with the realities of the effects of daily substance use, generally the people that they work with in the hospital are not still actively using drugs or don't have access to the substances they would normally use. It has been our experience that clinicians in the hospital appreciate knowing that there are community providers that they can have their patients follow up with post-discharge, and this sometimes makes them more willing to start people on medications, including long acting injections or community treatment orders if they know there is a psychiatrist and a treatment team that can continue these plans in the community. As street psychiatry teams working with patients often with no family involvement, we play an instrumental role in advocating for our patients and using our voices to paint a full picture of what our patients' lives look like, how their quality of life could be improved with treatment.

8.7 Grief and Managing Death on the Streets

People who are homeless are in a state of "survival mode" where their focus is typically on meeting immediate physical and emotional needs, and the complexity of processing grief may not be fully accessible or prioritized. However, the way people in survival mode manage grief can vary, and their coping strategies often reflect the need to simply get through the day or moment. It is important to be aware that grief is part of the story of how people become homeless, the loss of a sense of home, of social and family supports, of health are fundamentally a part of the stories of the people we work with. Often there are layers of grief that people experience. In our current toxic drug crisis people continue to lose their friends and family. Quite frankly, it never fails to surprise us to meet people where the number of losses they have experienced in a short time is completely overwhelming. Sometimes our own personal sense of grief is overwhelming as we count along the number of people we know together that we have lost.

Therefore, as clinicians it is important to be aware of the prominent role grief plays in our patient's lives and in their mental and emotional wellbeing. The following sections describe some ways people in survival mode might manage grief:

8.7.1 Emotional Numbing and Avoidance

In survival mode, emotional numbness can be a common coping mechanism. People may distance themselves from their emotions to avoid feeling overwhelmed. This might manifest as feeling detached, as in "shutting down" or emotionally "I want to cry but I can't." It's a protective mechanism that helps people manage the immediate crisis, but it can make it more difficult to grieve deeply.

As clinicians we may become frustrated with our patients around their unwillingness to talk about their emotions. Our patients describe their multiple losses, their trauma symptoms, their substance use to deal with these difficult feelings, and we desperately try and create a safe space to help explore these deep hurts. But if we are meeting with people on street corners, under bridges, in places of abject poverty, we need to be mindful that people aren't in a place where they can feel this deep hurt. It simply isn't safe for them to walk around in such a vulnerably emotional state. It is still important that we acknowledge our patient's grief, if we are aware of a recent loss they have experienced to let them know how sorry we are and to check in how they are doing. Ask about their coping mechanisms, if they are eating, sleeping, able to meet their basic needs, if their substance use has gone up or if they are having suicidal thoughts. Our patients may not be ready to do the heavy emotional work, this may not happen for years, but talking about grief, educating our patients about the normal ups and downs of grief, is helpful. Try to keep in mind, months down the road, about those significant losses in your patients' lives. This shows genuine care for your patient but also may help give them insight into some of the challenges they've been experiencing since that time and why.

Example: a person might suppress tears or avoid discussing their loss because they feel too overwhelmed or unable to handle the depth of their sadness. However, you notice that they seem to be using more substances since the recent overdose of a close friend.

8.7.2 Denial, Distraction, and Busyness

Denial and staying busy can be another way people in survival mode manage grief. The individual may not fully accept or process the reality of their loss because it feels too unbearable to confront. Denial helps create a buffer between the person and the emotional pain, allowing them to focus on more immediate, survival-related tasks. For those of our patients who have learned to survive since an early age by taking care of others, you may notice that they fall into a pattern, especially with grief, of focusing on other's pain during times of grief rather than their own.

Example: Even though your patient has just lost their long-term boyfriend from overdose while he lay beside her in bed, she is focused on taking care of everyone in the community who is sad, often seen comforting others about his loss, rather than being comforted herself.

8.7.3 Physical Symptoms of Stress

When in survival mode, grief may manifest more through physical symptoms, such as fatigue, insomnia, headaches, or a lack of appetite. These physical signs can be the body's way of responding to the stress and emotional strain, rather than through more overt expressions of sadness or mourning. People may focus on these physical symptoms, especially when they feel like they can't process their grief directly.

Example: Your patient tells you how she has been struggling with decreased energy for months and difficulty with sleep since her son died. When you try to talk with her about how she is coping with her son's death, rather than engaging around her feelings she keeps asking for help with her energy.

8.7.4 Overwhelming Emotional Bursts

While people in survival mode may suppress or avoid grief for a period, there are moments when the grief surfaces uncontrollably. These emotional outbursts may occur unexpectedly when a trigger surfaces or when the person has some space to process their emotions. These moments can feel intense, but they may also provide a release and an opportunity for healing. Part of being culturally sensitive is being aware that different cultures have very different norms around grief and what is expected. Be aware of your own biases or how people are "expected" to behave while they are grieving. Does your culture/community grieve in a very public, loud, expressive way? Are men allowed or expected to wail or cry? Do people show their grief in physical ways such as with what they wear or by public gestures? Think about these things also when thinking about how you and your team talk about grief, how we may pathologize normal grief reactions.

8.7.5 Connection to Support Systems

Even in survival mode, support from others can help people manage grief. While they may not be able to fully process their feelings, having a supportive network of family, friends, or professionals can offer a safe space for them to share when they are ready, or simply feel seen and understood. Our patients often talk about their "street family" as their main support, so be aware of who your patients rely on, who they sleep with outside, if the losses they have experienced are also shared by others in their community and if they are able to talk about these losses with their informal supports.

8.7.6 Long-Term Delayed Grief

For some individuals in survival mode, the intensity of grief might be postponed. While they may not actively grieve in the immediate aftermath of loss, the emotions could resurface later when they are in a less stressful situation, or when they feel more emotionally able to handle the grief. In this case, the grief process might be delayed but eventually needs to be fully addressed. Sometimes if we have known patients for years on the street, it can be quite powerful to see after they have moved into housing and experienced the safety and security of housing to hear our patients reflect on things that they may have experienced during the last few years and how tough these experiences/losses were. It is part of the privilege and therapeutic aspect of knowing people for a long time to be able to reflect about their relationship with people they have lost, to share in that loss with them, and to also talk about the growth and new relationships you have seen people form since that loss.

8.7.7 Grief Through Action

Sometimes people in survival mode manage grief by channeling their emotions into actions that honor the memory of their loved one or their loss. This could involve engaging in charitable activities, organizing memorial events, or taking steps to create a legacy. By focusing on positive actions, they may find a way to integrate the grief into their lives without feeling overwhelmed by it.

As health care professionals it certainly isn't in our job descriptions to create meaningful rituals for our patients to mark significant life events such as birthdays or funerals. Yet, many health and social services providing care to the homeless do make this an aspect of providing care. You may want to familiarize yourself with how the street organization and/or street community you are working with memorializes your patients, are there formal gatherings or informal gatherings? Is there an "overdose memorial site" in the city where you work? It is part of our job description to help connect patients to resources that empower them to grieve effectively. This helps you connect your patients with appropriate community resources and supports for grief. In the US, many homeless health organizations acknowledge and mourn the people's lives that were lost due to homelessness on the winter solstice. National Health Care for the Homeless Council encourages every HCH-funded federally qualified health center to hold a Homeless Person's Memorial Day on the solstice that includes reading the names of people who died while homeless during that year. In Pittsburgh, Jim Withers' organization created a Memorial Wall. Each year on the solstice, new plaques are placed on the wall with the names of the people who died literally on the streets. https://www.wesa.fm/identity-justice/2014-12-19/honoring-pittsburghs-homeless-who-died-in-2014

With the large amount of death that is seen on the streets due to the toxic drug crisis and oppressive social and health care systems, funerals and rituals feel in some ways like a political act. This person was here and by marking their life, we are not letting others forget it. Funerals serve as important community functions as well—they help individuals process grief, honor the deceased, and support the bereaved. We have also experienced that for our patient's families who often are impoverished themselves, or don't know how to memorialize their family member due to their complicated relationship/estrangement experiences, there is a profound sense of peace and belonging in being able to come together with their family member's chosen community to commemorate together who they were. Families need these "alternative" spaces of grieving. For staff and peer workers who have worked and been friends with patients for sometimes decades, having the space to grieve and commemorate the lives of people is important also for helping to acknowledge their grief and loss.

8.8 Post Death Team Debrief

This is a debrief tool that we use with staff after a client has passed in one of our programs.

> "We're looking to debrief in ways that honour connection, center our collective care, and are an enactment of our commitments to each other as coworkers. We begin by committing to connecting immediately following a traumatic event, co-regulating each other, and staying with connection to prevent further traumatizing each other. Vikki Reynolds—https://vimeo.com/269393114?embedded=true&source=video_title&owner=84891408"

- Introduction—who we all are
- Confidentiality
- Choice to share versus silence-respecting that some people will want to talk, some people will want. Not judging each other for how we react to these situations, what types of care we need.
- What do we know about the death? Do you have unanswered questions about the death or incident? Want to make sure people have the facts
- Memories/thoughts they have been having of person who died, how has the death impacted them, how do they see others around them reacting
- What do you need as an individual to cope? What does the team need? How have you coped with difficult things like this in the past?
- What hopes do you carry for your work, your role
- Closure-summary, validating, normalizing roles-reminder that peer support is always there. Making an agreement to check in with each other over the next few days-other staff who may be missing from debrief.
- Reminder about being kind to each other as surest way forward
- How can we honour the person who died?

Warning Signs of Compassion Fatigue Feelings of helplessness/powerlessness

- Reduced feelings of empathy and sensitivity
- Increased anxiety, sadness, anger and irritability—are people in your personal life or your colleagues finding you are a different person?
- Feeling overwhelmed/exhausted by work demands
- Feeling numb, disconnected, detached
- Loss of interest/enjoyment in activities you normally enjoy
- Difficulty concentrating/making decisions
- Not taking care of yourself
- Increased use of substances, gambling, food, sex as a form of escape/numbing

How can you Take care of Yourself in this work?

- Eating, going to the bathroom, connecting with colleagues
- Mindful practices of how you transition from work to home—when are you giving yourself space to process your day
- Breathing/meditation/mindfulness/self compassion
- Reach out to others
- Taking care of yourself—eating, sleeping, exercise, connection with others
- Reducing your trauma inputs

- Maintain your work/life balance!
- Focus on those things that you do have control over
- Find awareness of what restores and replenishes you

Stay clear with your career goals/why you are doing this work

8.9 Encampment Sweeps—Contributing to Chaos

Consider exploring Schwan et al.'s guide on mitigating the health effects of encampment sweeps at https://hpri.usc.edu/wp-content/uploads/2025/04/Mitigating-the-Health-Impacts-of-Encampment-Sweeps-in-California-Practice-Guide-1.pdf.

Across the western world there is increasing visibility and complexity of homelessness, including encampments, in not only urban areas but also in rural, remote, and small towns. There is a real lack of awareness of the lack of places for people to go, a lack of understanding of how much homelessness really has grown across both rural and urban spaces and what has contributed to this. Encampments are the latest expression of a homelessness crisis decades in the making. These encampments are a tragic result of cracks in the foundations of our housing, health, and social systems and are a public policy failure by successive multiple layers of government. A lack of intergovernmental cooperation and integration of effort, and insufficient supply of affordable housing have compounded matters [1].

As street clinicians working with people who live in encampments, we have a front row seat to the harshness of the conditions our patients encounter, the stigma and isolation they feel from the rest of society, and an opportunity to educate citizens, policymakers and our local governments about this issue. Our patients tell us they feel unsafe in emergency shelters and frankly we witness the violence in shelters where theft, crowding and violence are common. Sleeping in a shelter means no privacy or autonomy or ability to sleep with your partner, friends or your pet. Shelters also have rules around people's behavior and substance use and so patients who are the most ill and have the most complex health and social issues without access to appropriate health care supports end up outside. Even if people did want to sleep in a shelter, there just aren't enough spaces anymore. In rural and remote settings shelter infrastructure hasn't been developed yet. People sleep in encampments out of necessity [9].

Living in encampments is hard work. There is the matter of sleeping outside and depending on where you live and the climate, it can take a lot of effort to stay warm enough or cool enough. There is the matter of finding food and clothing. There is also the matter of being vigilant for "sweeps" or being reported to the authorities. Encampments have often been responded to with large police-led clearings through the execution of sweeps and threats of arrest. Research has shown that these types of clearings have negative health consequences but are expected actions by cities without massive investments in housing alternatives [23]. For example, a study conducted in Hawaii found that 47% of inhabitants lost their personal identification during sweeps, 43% lost clothing, 40% lost tents, 24% lost food, and 21% lost medicine. Thus, disrupting encampments take away the stability, security, community, and autonomy of encampment residents [10].

As street clinicians a couple of things for you to think about when considering encampments is how are you going to introduce yourself to people? Remember you are entering people's home, think of what it is like for you to have people come unannounced to your home. Are you always prepared to have them come in and enter your space? It may take several visits before people will trust you. By visiting encampments are you attracting public attention to them or making patients feel like they are at risk for a sweep?

People living in encampments are very much in survival mode so meeting basic needs is going to be the priority. People may be living with very serious and complex health issues and be more concerned about where they will sleep that night than getting their health attended to. What supplies are you bringing with you to help you be ready for anything and what local resources can you share with patients. Are the medications you are prescribing or suggesting in line with the patient's lifestyle? For example, if you are thinking of an antipsychotic patients may not want to take something that causes them to become sedated when they need to be hypervigilant for people stealing their belongings.

8.10 Transition to Supported Housing—Important Considerations

The transition to housing can be chaos-inducing for patients. It is a time of massive change, losses and gains. It takes a different skillset to survive on the street than living in housing. There are different social norms, different rules to follow, and different relationships to navigate. The move into housing can mean the loss of relationships with outreach workers and fellow people living on the streets depending on the rules around guests in housing. After living on the streets for many years our patients may have forgotten the skills needed to maintain housing, such as cooking, cleaning, and remembering to take out their garbage. Some of our patients who have been on the streets from a very young age have never had the opportunity to learn these skills at all. It takes time for people to learn these skills and in the meantime their housing can become at risk if the housing environment they are in does not provide supports or understand the difficulties patients may have with this transition. Patients may also really struggle with going from living outside where they could use substances freely to being inside, where they may no longer be allowed to use substances. The opposite also occurs where patients were not using outside and now are surrounded by other people in their housing who are using and the person living next door to them is the local drug dealer and they relapse.

Patients are often surprised at how difficult the transition to housing is. It is something that they have often waited for years with high expectations and a sense that once they got housed that a lot of problems in their life would be fixed. Unfortunately, we see that when difficulties arise, patients can have huge issues with their self-esteem, self-image and sense of worthiness of having a home.

Particularly patients with histories of trauma who have a deep sense of shame and underserving may sabotage relationships during this transitional time. It's important to be able to talk frankly with patients about their fears. The sudden isolation of having their own room versus communal shelter/encampment living can have repercussions for both substance use disorder and mental health. In some cases, phobias may arise, or individuals may have difficulties staying inside when they are used to sleeping outdoors. In addition, the large change in environment and daily routine can cause trauma histories to manifest in new ways. Something that we have encountered, and that the literature also supports is large number of patients struggle with hoarding. When sleeping outside patients are used to collecting everything for survival purposes.

8.10.1 What Types of Housing Exists and What Philosophies Do They Use

One of the most important elements of health care is access to housing, which protects people from the elements and from many other dangers and health risks associated with living on the streets. Research has shown that housing has a positive effect on both chronic and acute medical conditions, patient's ability to manage treatment and medications, access to mental health services and substance use treatment and overall quality of life. There are a lot of different housing models for people living with chronic physical health issues, mental health issues and substance use and these will look different depending on where you live, whether harm reduction services are allowed, and the funding/political will towards reducing homelessness. Two types of housing common in the homelessness literature are Housing First and permanent supportive housing.

Housing First is a human rights philosophy that everyone deserves a home and that there is no expectation of sobriety, treatment, behavioral stability, etc., before receiving a home. Housing is the first intervention and additional health and social supports are provided once a patient is placed in housing. Permanent supportive housing emphasizes long-term affordability with the provision of services, ideally an interdisciplinary model that promotes ongoing stability of mental and physical health, substance use and trauma. Housing delivery models can include single-site, scattered site, mixed populations and more.

8.10.2 What Successes Exist to Ease the Transition into Housing and to Mitigate Potential Harms of Moving into Housing

As mental health clinicians our expertise may not be housing but we play an important role in helping to facilitate the transition between living on the streets and being housed. These outcomes align with accumulating evidence that integrating health care services with housing programs enhances the likelihood that people who are homeless will successfully transition into shelters, interim housing, or permanent housing [11]. This is neither a simple, linear or quick thing to do and is quite complex. The important thing to keep in mind are the small wins, things like starting to take medication, engaging with a housing worker, are all small steps where our patients start to believe in the care we are providing, in their own abilities to create change. We carry the hope for our patients reminding them that they deserve these things and giving them the tools to go after what they desire [17].

Another important element to consider in the transition to housing is the transfer of harm reduction supports. Boston's Harm Reduction Housing Model notes six core principles which include harm reduction supply accessibility, colocated medical services, resident autonomy and privacy, resident safety and security, community promotion and transitional supports. Addressing risks related to substance use among unhoused populations is crucial for mitigating overdose risk and establishing housing stability [23]. For patients who are transitioning from a shelter where they may have had to hide their substance use, transitioning to a harm reduction housing model may require some adaptation and time to build trust. Peer support workers play an important role here in helping patients adapt to new norms around substance use.

8.10.3 What Are Unforeseen Consequences of Transitioning into Housing

Our experience at Ottawa Inner City Health Inc., has been that unfortunately while opening new harm reduction supportive housing units that we have lost significant amounts of people to overdose. Literature from both the USA and Canada indicates that housing environments are where the most fatal overdoses occur, largely because people are alone [7]. Even in supportive living environments, where substance users are housed together with supports, they are still sleeping in their own separate rooms. This is much different from the shelter environment or encampments where people are often sleeping together, carrying naloxone (Narcan), and the homeless community along with outreach/shelter staff are responding to overdoses and saving lives. In supportive housing, an important intervention to mitigate overdose risk is to build sense of community and looking out for each other. We've been very fortunate to see patients themselves become part of the solution; developing peer safety checks where they have scheduled times where they walk around the building knocking on people's door, carrying naloxone, and responding to overdoses. Patients find this intervention helpful as it feels less invasive than staff coming into their rooms and they trust co-patients to be less likely to give them too much naloxone and drive them into dope-sickness. The peers have really been empowered from becoming leaders in their community, having paid work, saving lives, doing meaningful activity and we have seen that this has driven them to become further educated. For example, our housing peers have asked to get CPR training to better respond to overdoses and have started a health advocacy group where they present on different common health issues.

Staff in our supportive housing units do safety checks on patients who are using, and patients can opt-in or opt-out of safety checks with education about the potential risks. Something else that we have adopted in our supportive housing units is overdose detection technology (ODTs). There are three categories of ODTs with varying practicality, privacy and invasiveness. Fixed location devices work as a form of communication between the person using drugs and support staff to provide privacy but assistance when necessary. Smartphone applications will alert the correct people to aid as long as the person using drugs keeps their phone nearby. Reverse motion technologies can be useful in business or hospital restrooms for instance, where there is high drug use. Wearable auto-injector technology is more invasive but carry's an extra layer of safety as the device literally injects naloxone into the individual [12]. Our experience in Ottawa has been that we needed peers to invest a lot of time and motivation with patients to get them invested in using the technology. Just like with any technology implementation change there must be buy in, education about the technology, teaching people how to use it and then motivation for ongoing use.

8.10.4 Methods of Helping Patients Stay Housed

Patients have identified that making the transition from the culture of street living to being housed is hard. Having to make adaptations to a new social environment, encountering feelings of disconnection and loneliness are common. If people having been living outside on their own and completely isolated having to relearn how to engage with people and deal with common sources of conflict of living with others is completely normal and overwhelming. Homeless patients have identified the importance of having support people that were emotionally consistent, authentic and reliable during the transition from homelessness to becoming housed [13]. For example, California's Healthcare in Action's success in supporting housing stability can be attributed to building trust between patients and health care providers. When homeless people receive compassionate, person-centered care from providers who understand their unique challenges, they feel supported and empowered to make positive changes in their lives [17]. Having supportive people provide gentle and slow hand-offs to new staff in housing units is also important. As support staff if we show our patients that we trust their new care providers, it will help our patients know that they can trust them too.

Housing was identified by patients as an opportunity to rebuild family relationships. Patients have also identified experiencing "housing guilt"; feeling bad about their street friends and family not having access to the same services as they have. This can become a risk to one's own housing status as we see clients attempt to house their friends and family with them in their bachelor apartment and get in trouble for their guests' behavior. It is important to be mindful that for people coming from certain cultural background this is particularly important. For example, our First Nations and Inuit patients in Canada have a strong sense of community and sharing their belongings is part of their cultural practices. Sharing housing is often a reason why we see our Indigenous patients become unhoused. We need to design housing policies that are culturally informed.

Many individuals living with chronic physical and/or mental illness, substance use and trauma histories experience difficulties chronically or episodically, meaning that they will live with these issues to a greater or lesser extent over their lifetime. A common misconception about supportive housing is that it is transitional but for our patients with profound cooccurring brain injuries, substance use, physical health challenges and mental health challenges supportive housing plays an important role in helping to optimize our patient's functioning. Adopting a recovery-oriented approach to how we work with patients is important. We need to be mindful that the functional challenges of our patient's illness that have contributed to them becoming homeless may remain and are important to keep in consideration during the transition to being housed. We need to help emphasize hope, our service user's natural support networks, that recovery is personal and nonlinear, and help our patients create meaningful lives despite living with challenges [13].

There is a still a lot about the transition into housing we don't know, particularly how to know who will or won't be successful and what type of barriers people have that we wouldn't account for. A high level of understanding and consciousness among care providers, plus a robust network of wraparound supports, is necessary to support people through the many challenges that arise when transitioning into housing. At the core of these supports should be an acknowledgment of the autonomy of the patient, and a trauma-informed commitment to supporting them, as they are ready to take steps to change their lives, improve their health, and return to planning and dreaming about their futures.

Street medicine teams may or may not have the ability to follow patients into their housing based on their funding and their mission. If a street medicine team is able to continue to follow a patient into housing, the team can be a positive support to help the patient manage this difficult transition. The hard part can then be as a team figuring out how long to remain connected to the patient or finding a primary care team to connect your patient to. If your street team is not able to remain connected to people once they enter housing, it's important to try and help identify a primary care team or supports that your patient will be able to access once they are in housing. Otherwise there are concerns that all the good work your patient and your team has done to get the patient housing ready will be derailed by the lack of access to appropriate supports.

8.11 End-of-Life Care for People with Profound Substance Use/Mental Illness

It should be noted that palliative care for the homeless is a whole other specialization so below we will just briefly summarize a few points to consider when working with those with profound substance use issues and/or mental illness that may put them at risk for increased mortality and morbidity. To clarify terms, palliative care aims to improve quality of life and relieve suffering of patients facing serious illness, as well as their family members, through a "whole-person" approach to care that provides early identification, assessment and treatment of pain, as well as addressing all other physical, psychosocial, and spiritual issues. Palliative care is holistic care offered in any setting to any person of any age living with serious illness. It includes a range of care providers including patient's unpaid caregivers [8]. End-of-life care (EOL) refers to care provided to those who are terminal and predicted to die within the near future [18]. Thinking about palliative care with our patients who are living with treatment refractory mental illnesses helps us to reflect with our patients and with ourselves about what quality of life looks like. What would these patients want for themselves? How does this change their outlook on life, their goals or decisions about their health and treatment?

Our patients have long histories of surviving things that other people wouldn't. They have witnessed many people in their social networks die and many have repeatedly been told they were going to die because of their "lifestyle." This creates a particular relationship with death among this community, on one hand death is "normalized," on the other hand there is such a strong sense of the will to survive. This is a particularly unique part of doing this work. I've witnessed many times physicians who are highly regarded in their field come and work on the street and be alarmed at a patient's health status. They've looked at me and said "Kim, this person is going to lose their leg" or "they are going to die, we need to do something." I share their concern for our patient's well-being, but I don't often carry the same fear that our patients won't make it, because repeatedly my patients have shocked me with their will to live and their resilience to live through things my white privileged suburban life wouldn't live through. When we tell our patients that we are concerned that they are going to die if they don't get this issue taken care of, it's not surprising that they don't react strongly. Often, it's only because of our relationship with patients and us not abusing/overusing this expression/overstating the risks that patient's will follow their own instinct about themselves and seek further care.

Some of our patients have severe and persistent mental illness (SPMI) which is therapy-refractory, despite being on high levels of medication, engaging with mental health clinicians, being hospitalized multiple times, they continue to suffer with significant mood swings, psychosis, flashbacks, etc. Some of our patients have such serious substance use disorders that despite going to treatment dozens of times, trying medications, utilizing different types of therapies, experiencing the health and social consequences of their addiction and a deep desire to stop, they cannot. The needs of these patients sometimes remain unmet by therapeutic interventions, and they are at high risk of receiving care that is inconsistent with their life goals. Scholarly discourse has recently begun to address the suitability of palliative care approaches targeted at enhancing quality of life for these patients but remains underdeveloped [20].

How do we as clinicians work with these patients, considering that there is a high likelihood that these patients will encounter death in the next several years? Literature indicates that reducing suffering and maintaining daily life functioning are rated as considerably more important by patients than impeding suicide and curing the underlying illness. There are still considerable reservations towards palliative care in the context of psychiatric illness, mainly because of the association with death and futility. I know for myself, I have seen a very chronically homeless people with complex physical health and psychiatric comorbidities be discharged from a psychiatric unit with very little done to help alleviate their symptoms or provide direction on future care. The patient was discharged with "palliative psychosis." I read this and I was fuming mad. This person was in their mid-30s and had suffered so intensely. They had just been housed in a supportive housing building and were getting some stability in their life. With no recommendations on discharge, this wasn't palliative care, this was giving up on them and acting like there wasn't anything else we could do for them. As clinicians doing our best to help this person regain some functioning and sense of "normalcy" this diagnosis felt like such a kick in the teeth to our sense of hope for this patient. I wanted this psychiatrist at the hospital to be willing to take on some extra risk to care for this patient, to give them doses of psychiatric meds you might not see in a first episode psychosis. We see with our patients that are using drugs and psychotic that we must give them doses of antipsychotics that are beyond the normal levels but that the benefits to their functioning and ability to live in the community outweigh the risk to their health and potential side effects.

Within the currently existing literature, three main symptoms have been commonly observed in palliative care in our patients: pain, dyspnea, and anxiety/agitation. Literature indicated that pain is reported in significantly higher levels in people who use substances. Moreover, chronic opioid users frequently experience opioid tolerance and opioid-induced hyper-algesia, contributing to increased pain sensitivity. It's important to be mindful that pain can also emerge in the context of withdrawal symptoms. In palliative and end-of-life care, unlike chronic pain, tapering or stabilizing of opioids is not the primary goal of care. Potential side effects of higher opioid doses, as fatigue, are balanced against pain as a symptom, ideally in a joint decision with the patient, and advance directives should include these considerations. As psychiatric clinicians working with people with significant histories of trauma, it is important to be mindful of how our patient's emotional pain may be contributing to their physical pain and what can be done to help with this. Our patients are often used to using substances to help alleviate both their physical and mental pain and as their conditions deteriorate it may make it harder for them to get the substances they need to cope. What pharmaceuticals can we use as alternatives to help minimize their dependence for their usual substances? How can we develop harm reduction policies and procedures that are in line with how people want to die? As clinicians working with people who use drugs as they pass, we need to be prepared to deal with high amounts of opioids and psychiatric comorbidities [14]. At our shelter-based hospice in Ottawa, there are therapy dogs, access to Indigenous traditional healing, Country Food for our Inuit patients (traditional Inuit food including game meats and fish—important both as a source of nutrition but also as a fundamental part of Inuit culture), peer workers, mental health professionals, and clergy who provide spiritual support to people as they near end of life [15].

As psychiatric clinicians, one of our biggest struggles in providing good palliative care is that our patient's social care needs often feel like they are out of our scope of practice. Addressing deficits in housing, food security, income, transportation and other social dimensions of health are an essential component of quality palliative care for patients. As well there is a significant struggle to get our patients the appropriate health services in the settings where they live. We see our patients have health services discontinued even when housed because of safety policies that prevent home care from being delivered in settings deemed risky (e.g., overcrowded, where cigarette smoke, drugs, or drug-use equipment are present, or where violent incidents had occurred). Stigmatization of substance use and mental health issues influence access to care. This often leads to our patients being moved (often into acute care) as their care needs increase or they approach end of life.

We know from working with our patients that they prefer to stay in their community as they approach EOL, surrounded by familiar providers and support people they trust. There are models of shelter-based hospices and outreach palliative care teams and in places where these aren't available we know that there are frontline staff and street medicine teams going "above and beyond" their job descriptions, including doing personal care and providing medications to help their beloved patients die in places where they feel most comfortable [18]. There is also an international end-of-life doula association interested in working with people who are homeless and dying: https://inelda.org/dying-unhoused/.

I struggle when someone is labelled as palliative because like the above case, it can still be incorrectly applied to indicate that the patient's care should be shifted to end-of-life care. The population of patients that I work with has incredible resiliency and can achieve satisfactory quality of life with proper palliative care despite their severe and persistent mental illness (SPMI) which is therapy-refractory. As a result, despite the underdeveloped evidence for palliative care in this context, consideration for management strategies to improve quality of life should be considered for patients living with SPMI as continuing with standard therapeutic interventions that are not meeting their treatment needs or shifting to end-of-life care are not comprehensive enough options to meet life and treatment goals of all patients.

While I am comforted that the team that I am working with is aware of the modern definition of palliative care and does not associate it with only end-of-life care, I think that it can help our teams put into context the difficult lives our patients have led and come to terms with hard ethical situations. Especially when working with patients with severe substance use and mental health conditions. For example, several years ago, we had a young man in his 30s in our managed alcohol program with schizoaffective disorder. He was a total sweetheart and everyone on our team and the other patients adored him. He had a lot of friends in the program and often helped accompany more frail patients to their medical appointments. He started to show signs of liver failure and many members of our team spoke with him about reducing his alcohol use to help prolong his life. He was afraid of dying but he was also accepting of his prognosis. I remember him telling me that he hadn't expected to live this long anyways, that his life had been so hard, and that he didn't want to give up one of the things in his life that helped make it worth living. As someone who had worked with him for many years and had seen how far he had come, I knew how much he had struggled and how much emotional pain he lived with. We helped him make amends with his family during that time as his health deteriorated. We were able to help the team come to terms with his decision to not stop drinking and he was able to do life and his death on his terms. By communicating with the team that we were focusing on his quality of life from a palliative care approach, it helped us collectively work towards meeting his goals of care.

References

1. Association of Municipalities of Ontario. Homeless encampments in Ontario: a municipal perspective. 2024. https://www.amo.on.ca/sites/default/files/assets/DOCUMENTS/Homelessness/2024/AMO_Homeless-Encampments-in-Ontario_2024-07-02.pdf. Accessed 3 Feb 2025.
2. Baldasseri E. Newsom signs ‘CARE Court’ plan, overhauling mental health care in California. 2022. https://www.kqed.org/news/11924117/governors-care-court-plan-passes-assembly-clearing-way-to-become-law. Accessed 4 Feb 2025.
3. Bernheim E. Why involuntary medical admission and treatment won’t solve homelessness. 2024. https://theconversation.com/why-involuntary-medical-admission-and-treatment-wont-solve-homelessness-243428. Accessed 5 Feb 2025.
4. Brown T. Unknown challenges a homeless person faces. 2025. https://regenbrampton.com/unknown-challenges-the-homeless-face/. Accessed 5 May 2025.
5. CBC News. What it’s like to be homeless in Toronto. 2020. https://www.youtube.com/watch?v=w-s1p5z_W5E. Accessed 7 May 2025.
6. Dembosky A, Templeton A, Feibel C. When homelessness and mental illness overlap, is forced treatment compassionate? 2023. https://www.npr.org/sections/health-shots/2023/03/31/1164281917/when-homelessness-and-mental-illness-overlap-is-compulsory-treatment-compassiona. Accessed 5 Feb 2025.
7. Fleming T, Boyd J, Chayama KL, Knight KR, McNeil R. Using alone at home: what’s missing in housing-based responses to the overdose crisis? Harm Reduct J. 2024;21:24. https://harmreductionjournal.biomedcentral.com/articles/10.1186/s12954-024-00933-y.
8. Government of Canada. Palliative care: overview. 2025. https://www.canada.ca/en/services/health/campaigns/palliative-care.html?utm_campaign=hc-sc-palliative-care-24-25&utm_source=ggl&utm_medium=sem&utm_content=ad-text_en&adv=2425-643200&utm_term=palliative+care&gad_source=1&gclid=EAIaIQobChMIw_6NwdDfiwMVmEf_AR28FyGpEAAYASAAEgJTFvD_BwE&gclsrc=aw.ds#a3. Accessed 6 Feb 2025.
9. Houle MJ. Yes, you should be angry about homeless encampments. 2024. https://ottawacitizen.com/opinion/houle-yes-you-should-be-angry-about-homeless-encampments. Accessed 5 Feb 2025.
10. Junejo S, Skinner S, Rankin S. No rest for the weary: why cities should embrace homeless encampments. 2016. https://ssrn.com/abstract=2776425 or https://doi.org/10.2139/ssrn.2776425. Accessed 7 Feb 2025.
11. Koh HK, Restuccia R. Housing as health. JAMA. 2018;319:12–3. https://jamanetwork.com/journals/jama/fullarticle/2667710.
12. Lombardi AR, Arya R, Rosen JG, Thompson E, Welwean R, Tardif J, Rich JD, Park JN. Overdose detection technologies to reduce solitary overdose deaths: a literature review. Int J Environ Res Public Health. 2023;20. https://www.mdpi.com/1660-4601/20/2/1230.
13. Marshall C, Gewurtz R, Barbic S, Roy L, Lysaght R, Ross C, Becker A, Cooke A, Kirsh B. Bridging the transition from homeless to housed: a social justice framework to guide the practice of occupational therapists. 2020. https://www.sjmhlab.com/publications. Accessed 7 Feb 2025.

14. Marti L, Hunerwadel E, Hut B, Christ SM, Daster F, Schettle M, Seiler A, Blum D, Hertler C. Characteristics and clinical challenges in patients with substance use disorder in palliative care-experience from a tertiary centre in a high-income country. BMC Palliat Care. 2024;23. https://doi.org/10.1186/s12904-024-01366-x.
15. Nunavut Food Security Coalition. Country Food. 2024. https://www.nunavutfoodsecurity.ca/en/country_food. Accessed 7 Feb 2025.
16. Smith GP. After 25 years of being homeless I learned theres one simple thing you can do to help. 2018. https://www.theguardian.com/books/2018/jun/25/after-25-years-of-being-homeless-i-learned-theres-one-simple-thing-you-can-do-to-help-gregory-p-smith. Accessed 5 May 2025.
17. Subaiya I, Kaska B. What we've learned after four years of operating street medicine. 2025. https://www.statnews.com/2025/01/24/homelessness-street-medicine-medical-van-scan-group-healthcare-in-action/. Accessed 7 Feb 2025.
18. Stajduhar KI, Mollison A, Giesbrecht M, McNeil R, Pauly B, Reimer-Kirkham S, Dosani N, Wallace B, Showler G, Meagher C, Kvakic K, Gleave D, Teal T, Rose C, Showler C, Rounds K. "Just too busy living in the moment and surviving": barriers to accessing health care for structurally vulnerably populations at end of life. BMC Palliat Care. 2019;18:11. https://bmc-palliatcare.biomedcentral.com/articles/10.1186/s12904-019-0396-7.
19. Tornabeane ML, Tornabeane AS. Four ways to limit use of force in care of persons experiencing homelessness. AMA J Ethics. 2021. https://journalofethics.ama-assn.org/article/four-ways-limit-use-force-care-persons-experiencing-homelessness/2021-11.
20. Trachsel M, Hodel MA, Irwin SA, Hoff P, Biller-Andorno N, Riese F. Acceptability of palliative care approaches for patients with severe and persistent mental illness: a survey of psychiatrists in Switzerland. BMC Psychiatry. 2019;11. https://pubmed.ncbi.nlm.nih.gov/30975122/.
21. Vantol V. Being homeless takes a lot of work. 2021. https://invisiblepeople.tv/being-homeless-takes-a-lot-of-work/#:~:text=Keeping%20track%20of%20belongings%20Homeless%20people%20don%27t,is%20trying%20to%20protect%20them%20from%20theft.
22. Wade R. The homeless problem, my personal perspective. 2010. https://homelesshub.ca/resource/homeless-problem-my-personal-perspective-roger-wade/. Accessed 5 May 2025.
23. Zaragoza S, Silcox J, Rapisardam S, Summers C, Case P, To C, Chatterjee A, Walley AY, Komaromy M, Green TC. Developing a comprehensive inventory to define harm reduction housing. Harm Reduct J. 2025;22. https://doi.org/10.1186/s12954-025-01156-5.

Creating and Running a Street Mental Health Team

9

9.1 Building Your Street Psychiatry Team

The work we do as mental health clinicians requires personal vulnerability. We build deep therapeutic alliances in relationships with our patients, we learn profound things about ourselves, and need to find ways of healing our wounds, and develop intimate bonds with our fellow street team members. Part of the core foundation of building a street mental health team is finding the right people to do the work. This work isn't for everyone, it takes a special kind of professional to be willing to go into the unstructured environments, to be outside, to not always have office space, and to be so flexible. This work is gritty and dirty and painful at times. It takes special people who are willing to go above and beyond, who are comfortable in working in the gray.

In our current health care labor crisis where there is so much work and so few health professionals, it becomes harder to find the "right" people who want to do this work. Important traits to think about when hiring are empathy, a strong sense of ethics and boundaries, ability to handle crisis, creativity, flexibility, teamwork, and solid clinical assessment skills. Sometimes as managers our work is to find people who have the heart and build up the skills, sometimes it's about taking staff with years of clinical experience and helping them gain their own footing in working in such autonomous environments. When we are building up street teams, we must be mindful of building up and nurturing the strengths and well-being of our staff.

When considering developing a street mental health team, key tenets of street care include integration, low barrier, being trauma-informed, harm reduction focused and reality based [8]. We need to continue to respond to our patients and their changing needs with novel and radical approaches. Working from a harm reduction lens helps clinicians focus on working with patients without judgment, discrimination, or requiring them to stop using substances as a condition of receiving support. It uses out-of-the-box solutions and strategies that attempt to address the significant harms that are caused by substance use, complex trauma histories, and poverty. Any strategies to address harm should be based on evidence-based

S. Hatcher et al., *Street Mental Health Handbook*,
https://doi.org/10.1007/978-3-032-00663-9_9

research, public health, and human rights. While abstinence-based approaches work for those who are ready to quit, harm reduction serves a largely overlooked and marginalized population.

Harm reduction recognizes the autonomy of our patients to make decisions that are best for them. Stigma can reduce the willingness of people living with an addiction to seek care. With a harm reduction and trauma-informed care lens we approach each patient with compassion and empathy. Substance use becomes a health issue, not a moral or criminal one. Our patient's personal goals become be the guiding factor for care.

Important harm reduction services your team may want to think about engaging in are education, handing out clean drug equipment, training both staff and patients on how to give Narcan, teaching safe injection techniques, organizing site material disposal, managed alcohol programs, and providing prescribed pharmaceutical grade-opioids to reduce the harms of the toxic drug supply.

As a team, you really need to think about the population you are serving and how you can meet your patients literally where they are. Does this mean you will travel by foot, by bike, by car, by bus? Keep in mind your patients have limited transportation and mobility, so you need to be carrying things to them. Plan to carry items like socks, underwear, snacks, water, wound care supplies bags, gloves, Narcan, bus tickets-you want to be prepared to face different care scenarios and meeting people's basic needs is a good way to help people trust you and get them to engage in care with you. Street clinicians' sense of professional dress is different from what you may encounter in your other clinical roles—as street clinicians we want to dress to face the elements that we are going to face that day and to be aware that the patients we are encountering are living in abject poverty-so dress comfortably, practically and simply.

9.2 Components of a Successful Team

The success of a mental health team hinges on several key factors that enable effective collaboration, communication, and care delivery. These factors create a supportive environment for both the team members and the individuals they serve, ensuring that comprehensive, patient-centered care is provided. Below are key elements that contribute to the success of a mental health team:

9.2.1 Clear Communication

Open, honest, and frequent communication is essential for effective teamwork. Team members need to share information, update each other on patient progress, and discuss treatment plans in a respectful, collaborative manner. This ensures that everyone involved in a patient's care is on the same page and working toward common goals.

- Regular Team Meetings: Scheduled meetings where team members can discuss cases, share insights, and make decisions together. These are important opportunities for creating a sense of "sharing the load together" as the work itself can sometimes be isolating. How are we sharing laughs together, the joy of the work? How are we sharing our sadness and grief?
- Does your mental health team meet alone or also with the medical team (if you have one)? How is your team integrating your knowledge of the patient from a mental health and substance use perspective with their medical information? At Inner City we are very fortunate to have on our different units a physical health nurse coordinator and a mental health nurse coordinator with collaborating physician/psychiatrist. In some environments, mental health teams and physical health teams can be very at odds with each other-who is the most responsible team for a patient who has diabetes type 1 and is psychotic and using crack and won't take their insulin because they believe it is poisoning them? A complex patient like this can cause a lot of division among a team unless you have a strong sense of needing each other and appreciating the strengths of each other's knowledge and perspective. At Inner City, we do weekly mental health team rounds where the mental health nurses and psychiatrist get together and talk about what is happening on our units, what concerns we have, who we need to see and then on another day we have a larger full team rounds where we discuss everyone and include physical health, mental health and substance use concerns.
- Effective Use of Technology: Secure platforms or systems for sharing patient information, making it easy for all team members to access relevant data. Where/how does your team chart? How does your team share quick tidbits of advice, communicate during the day to ensure safety for example?

9.2.2 Role Clarity and Defined Responsibilities

Each team member must understand their role and how it contributes to the overall care plan. Clear role definition minimizes confusion, overlap, and gaps in care. Knowing who is responsible for what enables team members to focus on their area of expertise while trusting others to handle their responsibilities. Think about what stage of development your team is at. If you are a newly developing street psychiatry team roles will be less clearly defined and there will be more gray. Hire people who have lots of previous experience and confidence in their clinical assessments skills and are willing to work with some risk. As your team gets bigger, more structure, policy/procedure will be required.

Collaboration is a key element of street work. Working with different disciples, being open to different perspectives, working to the strengths of partner organizations is how we give our patients the best care. Need to leave our ego aside and think about what is best for the patients. Consider how your team can find opportunities to switch to different roles as clinicians—housing vs. outreach, crisis vs. long-term engagement. This can help your team understand different perspectives and manage transitions from street to housing for example. This can also help promote staff wellness by switching up how much acute crisis staff are dealing with. Growth opportunities in and out of the organisation can allow clinicians to aim toward transferring into other positions and empower clinicians in their ability to deal with complex situations on their own.

9.2.3 Mutual Respect and Trust

A strong, positive team dynamic is built on trust and respect for each other's expertise, experiences, and perspectives. When team members trust each other, they are more likely to contribute openly, ask for support when needed, and remain focused on the patient's best interests. This work is hard, having a sense of team is really what makes this work manageable in the long term. As a manger, take the time to focus on your team's well-being, check in about shared values and goals, create opportunities for team members to get to know one another and have a sense of each other's values. Share in each other's small wins and losses. Make space and time for fun together. Build a strong sense of humour among your team based on compassion for each other and having each other's backs. This is an important element in helping make the work enjoyable, preventing burnout, and sharing knowledge, resources, and creativity together.

Team members should respect different professional backgrounds, ideas, and approaches to care. The homeless are a diverse bunch of people, having a diverse staff helps you respond to their needs. How do you engage your team, foster diversity and value voices that may not be heard as easily? Be cognisant of who carries power on your team, who shares information, and how your team make decisions about clinical care. Encourage team members to actively listen to each other to foster an inclusive environment.

9.2.4 Shared Goals and Vision

A successful street psychiatry team must be aligned in terms of the overall mission and objectives for patient care. When everyone shares the same vision for a patient's recovery or well-being, it helps prioritize the right interventions and outcomes.

- Patient-Centered Goals: The team's goals should be focused on the individual's needs, values, and preferences.
- Measurable Outcomes: Setting clear, measurable goals and tracking progress ensures that the team stays on track and keep goals realistic. Sometimes we want things to move more quickly than they do. Recovery takes a long time, and setbacks are to be expected. Help manage expectations and be realistic about the resources available.

9.2.5 Adequate Support and Supervision

Regular supervision, professional development, and ongoing support are critical for street mental health teams; this is an emotionally demanding environment. These tools ensure that staff members are not only equipped to handle their roles but also have the tools to cope with the stress of working in mental health. Team members should have access to supervision to discuss complex cases, get advice, and manage personal challenges. Renowned street therapist Vikki Reynolds notes "the therapists I work alongside most desire is to be of use to their patients…many therapists suffer from a cold fear in the belly that incompetence or a lack of knowing on their part may result in devastating consequences for patients…losing patients to suicide and violence death is a reality. Experiences of being overwhelmed are not uncommon. Job titles such as support worker, shelter worker, or addictions counsellor offer only thin descriptions of the complex demands of their work, and do not honour the magnitude of trauma, violence and exploitation that shape the identity of patients…in these contexts, therapists struggle to practice in line with their ethics, and to help patients' keep a fingerhold on their dignity" [6, p. 247].

Providing staff supervision is an important element of taking care of staff well-being and helping to translate the vision, mission and values of your organization into the clinical work of frontline staff. Clinical supervision offers the opportunity to develop staff in their clinical skills, debrief on elements of their work that they are struggling with (for example, a common question to ask is "who/what is taking up space in your head?"), help staff reflect on elements of their work that they may want to receive further education/skills development on, and overall helps both the staff and the clinical supervisor to reflect on patients, program development and ways to improve quality care for the patients we serve.

It's important to be mindful of how you want to provide supervision and who will be able to provide supervision. There may be different people in your organization that are part of your supervision process. Are you providing supervision to staff at all levels of your organization for example frontline providers, program managers, directors, and others? Do you have the capacity to provide one-on-one supervision and/or group supervision? Be mindful of where people are at in their careers as clinicians but also particularly in starting street work and their exposure to street life. For example, at Inner City when we have new mental health nurse coordinators orientating, I debrief with them daily and as they get more comfortable in their role this changes to weekly supervision sessions with ongoing on-call availability for crisis/new situations that arise. On top of this my coauthor Simon Hatcher provides monthly supervision to our nurses in a group format where we talk with each other around those people taking up a lot of space in our head.

Supervision of staff is based on relationship and rapport between supervisors and their staff. Vicki Reynolds eloquently refers to this as "supervision of solidarity" in which supervisors are working with frontline staff in solidarity towards doing just work in the face of oppressive contexts. It relies on building a strong relationship of reciprocity and cultural humility, of active listening and empathy for the hard work staff do every day. For clinical supervisors it is expected that you schedule supervision regularly and that you make the effort to show up. As supervisors working with staff who have experienced trauma, we need to treat our staff with the care and consistency we expect them to show our patients. Have a set date and time when you meet, prepare an agenda, have things you want to review, discuss support and professional needs, take the time to practice skills together and provide constructive/positive feedback (Lang & Platts, 2024, "personal conversation") [3].

9.2.6 Burnout Prevention

Teams should have strategies in place to prevent burnout and support self-care among staff. When we engage with different social service sectors interacting with street engaged people, whether that be shelter workers, outreach workers, health care providers, etc. we hear street-based organizations talk about struggling to recruit and retain staff because of burnout, precarity of employments (so often people start in this work on contract because new programs are started with only 1 year funding) and the very difficult nature of the work itself. The pandemic, the toxic drug crisis and the increasing rates of homelessness and negative political and social attention around these issues have only amplified these chronic concerns. For example, research indicates that on average, outreach workers conduct direct outreach services for 3 years. This turnover rate, symptomatic of the trauma, stress, and burnout that are inevitable parts of the job, indicates the need for outreach programs to have a built-in support system for staff which includes caring for outreach workers' well-being, career development opportunities, and providing evidence of their success through evaluation. There is a lack of research that has examined the turnover rate in psychiatrists, physicians, nurses, social workers and other professionals working on the streets however we have witnessed a high turnover among our collective teams [7].

Focusing on job satisfaction and emotional detachment can be developed as a means of inhibiting empathy bleed, where concern for others well-being inhibits a person's ability to care for themselves. A common strategy for institutionalizing individual well-being is to make accessing the services mandatory. An organization in Virginia requires its workers to access free monthly counselling from a Presbyterian Counseling Centre. Once a month, they are paid to attend a weekend activity of their choosing and have the rest of the weekend off. In San Francisco, outreach workers are required to employ an adapted "Healing the Healers" protocol and attend different self-care activities including Eastern medicine, group processing, and conversation with a mental health professional [10].

Individually as a clinician how do we manage burnout? We can't do this alone. Across organizations and across street teams, there is discussion about the need to create community around doing this work, around celebrating the joy and the grief in the work not alone, but together. The Grey Badgers, a group of frontline workers from London, Ontario suggest organizing a group of peers at your workplace to discuss your feelings with regularly, finding a way to support each other and continue in the work together. They encourage street clinicians and peers to regularly engage with their employers around employee wellness. Some other suggestions they have are to think about creating a sector-wide across agency buddy system so that everyone has someone they can check in with about difficult feelings 24/7. They also note the importance of vigils and recognizing those staff who no longer work in the field and gratitude for their service [8].

Vikki Reynolds in her work on compassion fatigue notes the importance of building a healthy team that supports each other by balancing work and play. A healthy team finds space for humour and space for being able to express grief together. As team managers it can be a tricky balance between wanting to take care of our staff and not becoming their therapists. Helping advocate for good benefits for your staff that include access to psychotherapy and body work helps give staff the appropriate clinical supports to keep doing this work. Across different frontline sectors-police, paramedics, firefighters, military and street work there is increasing research and development being done of programs to help prevent and treat vicarious trauma, recognizing that this is an inherent risk to our physical and psychiatric/ emotional well-being in doing the work.

9.2.7 Staff Education

As an organization, what is your orientation training like for staff? Do you regularly schedule staff trainings that help clinicians learn updated knowledge about issues they may confront on the streets? How are you getting staff trained to work with people who are experiencing homelessness? Are you teaching them about the values and philosophy that underpin the work your organization does as well as the clinical skills needed to do the work? As street-based organizations we also need to focus on how to retain experienced staff so that they can train others and contribute to team wellness/experience/knowledge base. Some things that have been found to be helpful include ongoing education provided by team members or experts outside of your organization, providing ample opportunities to learn aside experienced street clinicians and see how they tackle tough conversations and challenging clinical situations, and going to conferences where you get excited about the work (the Street Medicine Institute conference is great for example!).

9.2.8 Flexibility and Adaptability

Mental health care often requires a flexible approach, as patient needs can change over time, and challenges may arise unexpectedly. A successful team is adaptable, able to adjust to new circumstances, and open to revising treatment plans based on evolving needs.

- Adapting to Changing Needs: Whether the patient's condition improves or worsens, the team should be able to pivot and update the care approach accordingly.
- Problem-Solving Skills: A willingness to think creatively and collaborate on challenges ensures that obstacles do not hinder patient care.

9.2.9 Cultural Sensitivity and Inclusivity

A diverse mental health team is more likely to successfully serve a wide range of patients with varying backgrounds. Teams must be culturally competent, aware of the unique challenges faced by individuals from different communities, and sensitive to the stigma that may exist around mental health care.

- Cultural Competence Training: Providing team members with ongoing training in cultural sensitivity helps ensure that care is respectful and tailored to diverse patients.
- Respect for Patient Autonomy: Recognizing and respecting the cultural values, preferences, and needs of patients enhances their comfort and engagement in treatment. Dr. Turnbull, the former medical director of Inner City, would comment that sometimes what clients can't tell us what they want/need but their actions tell us a lot. For example if we keep sending people to hospital for a complex medical issue with the intention of giving our patients equitable access to appropriate care and they keep leaving against medical advice. Sometimes we can get caught up in *our* worry about the patient not getting the level of care that they deserve, rather than respecting that the hospital isn't our patient's desired place to be, that they aren't getting their needs met in hospital and maybe this means we need to find a way to do our best to meet their needs in the community

9.2.10 Leadership and Team Management

Strong leadership is key to guiding the mental health team through challenges, ensuring that everyone remains motivated, and promoting a positive, collaborative environment. Effective leaders provide direction, facilitate discussions, and resolve conflicts, helping the team stay focused and unified.

- Leadership with Emotional Intelligence: A leader who is empathetic, supportive, and can manage conflicts helps maintain a cohesive team.
- Empowerment: Encouraging team members to take initiative, voice concerns, and contribute ideas fosters a sense of ownership and engagement.
- After the opioid crisis, there is a very strong sense of community trauma amidst organizations and their workers. How do we as leaders, who may carry our own trauma and grief, help build/maintain healthy organizations? Are we sorting through our own trauma and burnout and, doing the work of taking care of ourselves? So often with the incredible pressures of the work, clinicians, and

organizational leaders feel this strong sense to keep going, to keep pushing through for the sake of others. How do we lead by example?

9.2.11 Ongoing Evaluation and Feedback

Successful teams regularly assess their performance and the effectiveness of their approaches. Constructive feedback and evaluation allow for continuous improvement, helping teams identify areas of strength and those needing improvement.

- Regular Reviews: Continuous evaluation of team processes, communication, and treatment outcomes helps refine practices and enhance care delivery.
- Feedback Loops: A culture of feedback allows staff to improve their practices while ensuring patients' needs are being met effectively.
- Outreach work is fundamentally driven by a need to demonstrate empathy. However, as demonstrated by the average length of work, a person's ability to internally motivate themselves is limited. Organizations in Oakland and San Francisco found that by demonstrating the objective efficacy of their outreach work, protective factors such as job satisfaction and team cohesion were increased. For example, evaluators found that the pattern of outreach service was inversely related to crime in an East Oakland hotspot; an increase in outreach services was followed by declines in crime, and decreases in outreach services were followed by increases in crime. Furthermore, in a West Oakland hotspot, evaluators found that an intensification of outreach services in the month of March appeared to reduce crime in April and May [10].

In summary, a mental health team's success is largely determined by effective communication, mutual respect, clearly defined roles, shared goals, and a collaborative, flexible approach to care. By supporting each other professionally and emotionally, maintaining focus on patient-centered care, and adapting to the needs of both staff and patients, a mental health team can deliver high-quality, comprehensive treatment.

9.3 The Role of Medical Directives and Staff Mix

Our patients live in a world of crisis and when they reach out for health care, they want to be assured that they will get what they need in a timely fashion. Medical directives may be a useful tool for your team to consider to be able to reach more patients more acutely depending on your staff mix. For example, if you are a team that has less physician/psychiatrists and lots of experienced nurses, medical directives can enable your team to provide access to timely care and helps to meet patients in spaces where they are most comfortable. If you are thinking of using medical directives as a team, be aware of your Specialized College's practice guidelines/standards as this will be different depending on what state/province you practice in.

Medical directives are a prescription for certain procedures, treatments or interventions that nurses may fulfill or perform, for a range of patients, when certain clinical conditions are met. A medical directive identifies the specific condition, diagnostic intervention, procedure, treatment, and specific clinical circumstance which must exist before a directive can be implemented. They should also include contraindications for implementing the procedure. Medical directives need to clearly identify what physician is authorizing the medical directive and what nursing staff are authorized to use the medical directive.

It is a responsibility and privilege to provide care that is outside a nurse's normally defined scope of practice as a nurse. It requires a considerable level of trust and rapport between physicians and nurses and important care needs to be taken to ensure both nurses and physicians involved are comfortable with the arrangement. Organizations utilizing medical directives among their clinical team need to make sure that their nurses have the level of expertise, experience, maturity, and training to be able to utilize medical directives appropriately.

Street nurses need to feel empowered to use their intuition, community relationships, knowledge of the working environment and staff, in the programs they help to run. Medical directives may help your clinical team provide care in a consistent fashion according to best practices across different work environments. As street clinicians who are going out into the community, often alone or in pairs, having established protocols of how to provide care for certain common conditions is helpful for standardizing care and creating a unified approach across a team. Medical directives can be used as part of staff training programs, helping new or less experienced team members understand standard procedures and expectations. These directives serve as a reference point, helping staff feel confident in their roles and ensuring continuity in care as staff turnover occurs. Medical directives should be flexible documents that can be updated or revised as new research, practices, or regulations emerge. This adaptability helps the team stay up to date with the latest evidence-based practices and ensures that care continues to be relevant and effective.

At Ottawa Inner City Health Inc., medical directives were created initially when the team was very small, consisting of an internal medicine physician and a registered nurse. The physician was not available to see patients everyday; however, the nurse was in the shelter visiting patients and coming upon situations that needed care urgently. Our first nurse at Inner City was confident and had a lot of previous experience and a close relationship with our physician, who in turn had a lot of confidence in her and her ability to manage conditions. Together, they set out directives to help manage certain common conditions that were seen in the shelter-immunizations, TB screening, ordering BW, chest X-rays, treatments for abscesses, pneumonia, COPD, etc. When we had a mental health nurse practitioner join the team, medical directives extended to incorporate acute agitation, insomnia, and psychosis NOS. Our experience in having these medical directives was profound, it allowed us to treat patients with acute conditions that needed care and refused to go elsewhere for care. Medical directives helped make care patient-centered and it helped prevent hospitalizations. Our physician would round with nurses biweekly and follow up with complex cases. Often the most difficult part of giving good care to our patients is just finding them and finding them at a time when they are available to receive care. Our experience is that despite only having physician presence once or twice a week, our nurses who are in the shelter daily can manage a lot of clinical conditions.

9.4 Scope

Partnering with local universities and their medical, nursing, social work, occupational therapy, etc. programs is an important way to help students gain an understanding of the homeless population, the barriers they encounter accessing health care and the role street clinicians can play in helping improve health outcomes. Even if students don't plan to do street work when they graduate, having the opportunity to work with street teams that are passionate about improving equity can have a dramatic impact on students' sense of their role and the potential to improve trainee attitudes towards people experiencing homeless.

Partnering with local universities and colleges can be a creative way for your organization to recruit new staff and reduce stigma. We have heard from a lot of students of how working in a harm reduction community organization gave them a very different perspective of our patients but also what is possible in terms of different ways of providing care. They note the themes of social justice they encounter and passion that is sparked for advocating for underserved populations in their careers. Street Psychiatry experiences have been implemented at several health professions training programs and existing educational offerings across the United States and Canada [4].

9.5 Funding

There are more than 84 structured street medicine practices around the world, and these organizations are sparsely funded by institutions such as hospitals, universities, departments of public health, nonprofit organizations, and state/provincial and municipal governments (Worth, 2012). Street medicine leaders describe needing creativity and partnership as main values to help create funding for new street psychiatry teams. In the United States, the Health Resources and Services Administration funds programs and approximately 9% of HRSA's $2 billion annual budget is appropriated to health care for the homeless. In talking with street physicians and street psychiatrists, there is skepticism about billing as a sustainable option for funding homelessness services and billing can be laborious from a paperwork perspective as well.

There are multiple models of funding for street teams but having a stable source of income is essential. As well, consider how your organization will evaluate economic, health, and social outcomes as these are all important considerations for funders and making the case for what your organization is doing. Many street teams have multiple funders, sometimes including not-for-profit organizations such as the shelters who have a shared mission of serving the homeless population.

The USC Street Medicine team created a toolkit that may be helpful to your organization when considering starting up a street psychiatry team [11].

Canadian Example-Dr. Jeffrey Turnbull, MD and Wendy Muckle, RN, BScN, MHA, CM, Founders of Ottawa Inner City Health Inc.

Before Jeff and Wendy started Ottawa Inner City Health Inc. (OICH) they had established themselves as clinical leaders, humanitarians, and experts in program development with marginalized populations. They both had experience doing clinical work and program development in developing countries and a passion for working with the most vulnerable. In addition to being a specialist in internal medicine, Jeff was the Department Chair of Medicine at The Ottawa Hospital and University of Ottawa from July 2001 to June 2008, a position he later left to take on the role of Chief of Staff. Wendy was the medical director of Sandy Hill Community Health Centre at the time and had previously worked at the City of Ottawa with the homelessness team and from this job had lots of connections at the local homeless shelters. Wendy left a very secure job to take a leap of faith in starting Inner City. Both Jeff and Wendy were comfortable with taking risk at this point in their careers and were excited by the prospects of building a team who was motivated to deliver care differently to the homeless. They loved building intimate relationships with patients and gaining their input on how to design programs, and debating between themselves, with patients, and with partner organizations about how they wanted to design programs to make them the most patient-centered, efficient and unique.

Jeff and Wendy note how persistent they had to be in the beginning, how much they had to have a belief in themselves and their ability to create change for the most marginalized. They both had lots of career opportunities and Jeff noted there was many times that they could have just backed out, but "if it's the right thing to do, and the right way to do it…we had to be persistent". Jeff and Wendy both noted that at the time, they were also personally struck by the human suffering they were witnessing both internationally and locally with the HIV/AIDs crisis. In Ottawa, people with HIV/AIDS were literally dying on the streets in horrible conditions and "we couldn't abandon them." Wendy spoke about bringing staff from the provincial ministry down to the shelters to witness the work that they were doing and to look into the eyes of the patients they were working with. One of the ministry people cried as they witnessed a patient use their only quarter to pay for Jeff and Wendy's parking; this was an opportunity for people in power to really connect with the humanity of our patients and witness the generosity of our patients in real time.

In 2001 OICH received 3 years of Human Resources Development Canada (federal) funding. It was very difficult to get this federal funding switched over to provincial funding (health care is usually funded by provincial government). This was a pilot project with an evaluation component at the end of the funding which meant that they had to follow the plan and show that within 3 years the program had created meaningful outcomes in their patients' health.

Two significant challenges emerged during the early days of the pilot project. First, the Federal department which was providing funding was deeply impacted by political scandal making it almost impossible to pass funds in a timely manner. As a result, the pilot project which was scheduled to run for 3 years only had 2 years of operating funding due to multiple delays in releasing money. As well, one of the main partners, the Salvation Army, was undergoing a process of harmonizing its programs and approaches on a national level. This made getting permission to introduce a harm reduction program, during what was at the time an abstinence-based shelter program, extremely challenging. However, despite significant reservations and complex decision-making processes, ultimately, the senior leadership of the Salvation Army took an enormous leap of faith due to their desire to help vulnerable populations and threw their support behind Inner City Health. While frustrating at the time, this process yielded an understanding that partnership could mean that while we shared the same values, how they were operationalized could vary from one organization to the next which is a principle that has supported innovation.

After receiving the initial funding from the Federal government, they encountered a lot of difficulties in receiving funding from the provincial government, which normally funds health care. A lot of this difficulty was political, even though their program had shown success, the provincial government did not appreciate being told by the federal government provinces what to do and was resentful of having to pick up the tab for something that they didn't start or want and as a result, bureaucrats tried to stop OICH from continuing. Jeff and Wendy persisted in advocating and their community partners backed them up. CEOs of several of the local homeless shelters advocated to the province that they needed to fund OICH. Ultimately it was Jeff and Wendy's close relationship with The Ottawa Hospital that made a world of difference. The CEO of the Ottawa Hospital told provincial leaders that if OICH closed it could collapse their system in 1 day. OICH was on the verge of being shut down because of a lack of funding but the Ottawa Hospital ended up loaning OICH money and the province told them they would pay them back, they did but never did end up paying the interest on the loan. Jeff noted that years later the provincial minister who was ultimately responsible for funding OICH came up to him said how happy they were that they had funded the project.

Ultimately OICH received funding through the institutional branch, then through the mental health branch, then we got funded as a community health centre and that stuck, along with different funding streams. The Victoria Order of Nurses (VON), now Carefor, had been hiring personal support workers for 100 years so OICH partnered with them to provide personal support services in the shelter. Ottawa Public Health did a lot to support OICH especially when it came to providing preventative care and vaccines. The Ottawa Hospital has remained an important partner. Initially mental health services were outside the scope of what OICH was allowed to provide. This was because the province had funded a new program (implemented in 2 phases) which was going to empty the shelters of people with mental illness. This was the beginning of the intensive case management programs and Canadian Mental Health Association outreach services. This meant that we were not able to provide mental health care to people at our shelter-based medical unit, they had to be referred for a physical health reason only initially. When our partner organizations saw how quickly people who had been homeless for a long time got housed once treated for their mental health there was advocacy from the mental health sector to allow us to open to mental health referrals. Ultimately our partner organization The Royal Ottawa funded a nurse practitioner to provide psychiatric care in our programs and that was the beginning of OICH becoming an integrated physical, psychiatric and substance use service provider (Muckle and Turnbull, 2025, "personal conversation").

Jeff was familiar with medical directives from his work at The Ottawa Hospital, knew his availability to see patients was limited, and was very confident in the nursing abilities of Wendy and Louise who was our first nurse coordinator. Both Wendy and Jeff felt very strongly that to be patient-centered that we needed to have a nursing led organization. They felt that it was necessary to have nurses who could be in the shelters daily, becoming a familiar face for both patients and staff to build relationships and trust with. They had seen in other places that were very physician focused where there were locum physicians coming into shelters for only weeks at a time that there had been concerns expressed by both patients and partner organizations that there was no opportunity to build trust and relationship, no follow through, and so a lot of the most challenging patients weren't getting seen or were falling through the cracks. They saw physicians wanting to work patients up for health issues that weren't acutely urgent to the patients, they weren't their pressing need at the time. There was a mismatch between what the patients were looking for help with and the staff available to help them. Inner City found that using nurses with medical directives made more sense for what they were looking to do. Inner City also only got money for nursing from the government, we were expected to bill for Jeff's time. This didn't work particularly well because so many patients didn't have health cards, thankfully Jeff was employed in other places and didn't need the income from Inner City. In the beginning Jeff would check in with the nurses at the end of every day to go over prescriptions before the nurses sent the prescriptions to pharmacy. After several months Jeff wasn't calling into the check in every day anymore as he was feeling very confident in the nurse's decisions around patient care. This was the evolution of OICH becoming a nursing led team, and from here OICH began a progression of downloading responsibility from physician to nurses to personal supports workers and shelter staff to give our patients' care in the settings where they were most comfortable to receive it.

American Example—Eileen Reilly, MD, Boston Healthcare for the Homeless

Eileen is a beloved member of the Boston Healthcare for the Homeless Program's (BHCHP) team and an esteemed psychiatrist. Eileen was 26 when she cofounded Women's Lunch Place, a day shelter for women to go during the day. In 1986 she left the organization to go to medical school. Eileen worked as a psychiatry resident in her third and fourth year with Worchester Healthcare for the Homeless and then continued to work with this team as an Attending Physician for 3 years. She then went to Boston to work at Massachusetts Mental Health Centre. In 1998 she was hired by the Department of Mental Health to work in four homeless shelters before she joined the BHCHP Street team.

Eileen's heart and work is invested in the relationships she has built with people on the streets. She has returned to her day shelter as a psychiatrist in the summer of 2023. Those who work with Eileen comment on her knowledge of the population, her empathy, her ability to see the strengths in those she cares for, and the joy she has in spending time and getting to know her patients as people [2].

Boston Health Care for the Homeless Street Team was founded in 1985 when it first began caring in medical clinics and on the streets for individuals experiencing homelessness. Earlier that year, the city of Boston had a received a grant from the Robert Wood Johnson Foundation to create a Health Care for the Homeless program. A committee, led by the then-Boston Mayor Raymond L. Flynn and composed of the city's hospitals and homeless advocates, was tasked with creating a charter for this new program, with a mandate to end the existing fragmented state of medicine for this marginalized population by providing continuity of high-quality health care from street and shelter to hospital to respite care to home. The grant required a medical doctor to manage the care at BHCHP. Dr. Jim O'Connell joined that same year as the founding physician of BHCHP, having graduated from Harvard Medical School and recently completed an internal medicine residency at Massachusetts General Hospital. As a fully credentialed physician at Massachusetts General Hospital, Dr. O'Connell began a tradition of BHCHP clinicians being credentialed at either Massachusetts General Hospital or Boston Medical Center, thereby assuring the goal of continuity of care for our patients within the hospitals.

During that first winter of 1985, the number of people dying on the streets led the Massachusetts' Department of Public Health to fund an overnight van. Dr. O'Connell joined the van staff two nights each week to comb the streets of Boston seeking to engage "rough sleepers"—those sleeping on street corners, under bridges, down back alleys—by offering sandwiches, hot soup, blankets, clothing, medical care, a smiling face, and a consistent and nonjudgmental presence. BHCHP's street team continues to walk the streets of Boston and to be the medical presence on the overnight van, seeking out individuals whose struggle to survive each day makes access to our shelter and hospital clinics difficult while also making house calls to newly housed patients to continue their care and advocacy.

In 2002, BHCHP was notified about a national project by SAMSA joining together the Boston Health Care for the Homeless Program with the Massachusetts Mental Health Centre (a MA Department of Mental Health clinic) and submitted a proposal for a psychiatrist to work with primary care on the (already established) Boston Health Care for the Homeless Program street team to provide integrated care for unsheltered homeless persons. The proposal was accepted by SAMSA and BHCHP received 3 years of funding for a part-time psychiatrist and a part-time psychiatric social worker.

Eileen's presence had an immediate effect on improving the care for street patients. When the project ended, MA Department of Mental Health agreed to continue funding her position. Eileen feels very passionately about her work and that having psychiatry as part of street medicine is a crucial element in helping very mentally ill patients move into housing and improve their quality of life.

9.6 The Role of Peer Support Workers

Our patients tell us, and the research agrees, that peer support workers are an important element in improving care delivery, promoting recovery, reducing death, and advancing the quality of life of people who use drugs [1]. The experiences of homelessness, substance use, poverty, discrimination, and mental illness are all profoundly isolating and carry so much stigma. Peer support workers help bridge this sense of isolation by connecting our patients to people who have faced similar challenges to them. These relationships are validating, provide intimacy, and tools for survival that we as clinicians can't provide. Having peer support workers on your street health team is an important resource to help clinicians literally find those who need your help the most. Peer support workers help bridge the gap in understanding between us as clinicians who may have grown up in quite privileged circumstances and our patients, helping build bridges in trust, language and experience that enhances the quality of care for our patients [9].

Peer support workers are now being utilized in a variety of different settings and situations to help engage street involved people including delivering peer recovery coaching, patient advocacy, accompaniment to medical appointments, and facilitating groups focused on wellness and recovery [1]. Our experience at Inner City of incorporating peer workers is that it profoundly changed our ability to connect with our patients and help our patients feel understood. Our peer workers play a vital role in helping advocate for our patients when they take them to medical appointments and frankly some of our patients just wouldn't go to those medical appointments without a peer that they know and trust to accompany them. Our peers also play huge roles in our safe injection site by reversing overdoses and engaging with people around their substance use, their safety, what supports they need, and helping to bridge connections between patients and health care providers. We've also seen our peer workers play profound roles in helping create community when we start new supportive housing buildings by teaching patients how to respond to overdoses and use overdose technology, handing out safe drug equipment, engaging with patients about the stressors of moving from the street into housing and helping them to navigate these.

When working with peer support workers, be mindful of your power dynamic. Be respectful of their knowledge and experience. Be thoughtful about the toll the work of being a peer support worker takes on people, if this work is hard for us as clinicians who have close relationships with our patients, imagine what it is like for peer support workers to witness the pain and trauma that their close friends are going through. Peer support workers help keep the work that we do real for us, so they may expose us to uncomfortable truths about ourselves, making us aware of times our way of interacting with patients is oppressive or comes off in a way we don't want it to. Maybe we aren't centering our patient's experience as much as our own comfort. Despite doing the important work of literally keeping people alive, peer workers are often in precarious financial and housing situations themselves. Their work can be precarious to their own recovery and health and special supports are needed to help aid them in doing this work. As organizations employing peer workers, street medicine teams need to continue to advocate for better pay, benefits and recognition for the role peer workers play in helping improve access to care for marginalized populations [5].

9.7 Advocacy

So much of our work is advocacy and education. The rights of our patients to exist, to have homes, food, and basic human rights. If you are interested in working with more marginalized populations, if you have an interest in social justice, this work really provides the opportunity to learn the different ways health care providers can be involved in advocacy. As clinicians providing frontline care to patients, we do advocacy work every day in our interactions with paramedics, police, emergency rooms, family doctors, helping patients gain I.D., etc. We are always having to help explain to others in more traditional health care settings about the specific needs homeless people encounter. Be prepared that even in settings where you might expect people to have a better understanding of our population, particularly addiction and mental health settings, that you will still need to advocate to help people think about the challenges people without homes face. Be prepared to experience stigma as a clinician devoted to caring for this population. As a nurse it has been my experience that I wasn't taken very seriously by people unless I said the name of the doctor I was working with (who at the time happened to be heading the Canadian Physician's Association). One of the things I am most proud about with my time spent being a street nurse is the strong voice I have found within myself. When I first started if someone at the hospital told me something I didn't agree with about my patient, I wouldn't argue. But as time has gone on, I have found the courage to stand up and speak up for my patients and myself. Our voices matter. It makes me proud that I can stand up for my patients and articulate myself in an assertive manner where I get listened to, where I can hear the clinician on the other end of the line maybe grappling with a different way of looking at things. I have found it necessary at times to do this in person rather than on the phone with complex patients. Making my presence known at the hospital, making it very clear that even if this patient doesn't have family, they have care providers who care enough to come in. I've seen this make a difference not only for my relationship with my patients and their trust in me, but also for the trajectory of patient's care where care becomes provided in a way that is more in line with who our patients are and how they live their lives.

At Inner City some of the ways we have clinicians involved in advocacy and education is by training other professionals. For example, at times nurses have done training with paramedics and police officers about how to engage with our patients. After one traumatic incident where a police officer was very rough with one of our female Inuit patients, members of our nursing team did an education session for the police on working with women with previous experiences of trauma. Out of an awful event came education, and from this our nursing teams and some of our women involved in sex work developed positive relationships with a small team of police officers involved in human trafficking.

The work we do is political. Especially now. Part of the joy of this work has always been having a very real sense of how political policy impacts who we see on the street. However, in today's political and social climate where there is more discussion of the toxic drug crisis and homelessness in the news, often with a very negative take, it feels increasingly harder to do this work. The science of these issues often gets ignored. Often, we work in landscapes where we are seeing issues that haven't been researched before, and we must find new and creative ways to solve complex problems. As street clinicians be prepare to be considered an expert by local media outlets and politicians on these types of topics. Sometimes getting media attention can be good for funding, on the other hand when harm reduction work is getting a lot of negative political attention, having a low profile in the media may be best for your organization. When and how to be an advocate can take some savvy and lots of us have had times where our quotes have been taken out of context. Advocacy and our interactions with the media remain a tricky balancing act.

Advocacy often must be done at multiple systemic points; our work is complicated. Creating new programs or supportive housing may involve multiple layers of government including municipal, provincial and federal in Canada or city, state, and country in America and across different sectors-health, housing, legal, financial, etc. Think about how to translate your clinical experience and research along with patient stories into a narrative. You will need to become quite adept at trying to figure out your spin, how will you use the human story, touch on the financial impact of this intervention, the health outcomes, etc.

References

1. Ashford RD, Curtis B, Brown AM. Peer-delivered harm reduction and recovery support services: initial evaluation from a hybrid recovery community drop-in center and syringe exchange program. Harm Reduct J. 2018;15. https://harmreductionjournal.biomedcentral.com/articles/10.1186/s12954-018-0258-2.
2. Jolicouer L. 2025. https://www.wbur.org/news/2025/04/16/womens-lunch-place-shelter-boston-eileen-reilly-mental-health. Accessed 5 May 2025.
3. Lang D, Platts J. CMHA Ottawa model of clinical supervision. 2023.
4. Lo E, Balasuriya L, Steiner JL. A street psychiatry rotation for medical trainees: humanizing the care of people experiencing homelessness. Educ Case Rep. 2022;46:248–53.
5. Mamdani Z, McKenzie S, Pauly B, Cameron F, Conway-Brown J, Edwards D, Howell A, Scott T, Seguin R, Woodrow P, Buxton JA. "Running myself ragged": stressors faced by peer workers in overdose response settings. Harm Reduct J. 2021;18. https://harmreductionjournal.biomedcentral.com/articles/10.1186/s12954-020-004491.
6. Nolan S, Kelian S, Kerr T, Young S, Malmgren I, Ghafari C, Harrison S, Wood E, Lysyshyn M, Holliday E. Harm reduction in the hospital: an overdose prevention site at a Canadian Hospital. Drug Alcohol Depend. 2022;239:109608. https://www.sciencedirect.com/science/article/abs/pii/S0376871622003453.
7. Reynolds V. A supervision of solidarity. Can J Couns. 2010;44:246–57. https://cjc-rcc.ucalgary.ca/article/view/59283/44708.
8. Schoenberger SF, Cummins ER, Carroll JJ, et al. "Wanna cry this out real quick?": an examination of secondary traumatic stress risk and resilience among post-overdose outreach staff in Massachusetts. Harm Reduct J. 2024;21. https://doi.org/10.1186/s12954-024-00975-2.

9. Subaiya I, Kaska B. What we've learned after four years of operating street medicine. 2025. https://www.statnews.com/2025/01/24/homelessness-street-medicine-medical-van-scan-group-healthcare-in-action/. Accessed 7 Feb 2025.
10. The Gray Badgers. It's like working in a war zone-presentation. 2021.
11. USC Street Medicine & Center for Health Care Strategies. Financial planning for street medicine providers in California. 2024. https://www.chcs.org/media/Financing-Street-Medicine-Programs-in-California-Toolkit-2024-Update.pdf.

Psychosocial Interventions 10

This chapter reviews different treatments and approaches that have been used with people who are homeless and which can be generally included under the heading of psychotherapy. It also includes interventions which come under the heading of psychosocial such as Housing First and improving the discharge of people who are homeless from hospital.

Delivering psychotherapy to people who are homeless is often portrayed as fraught with challenges and best avoided. While classic weekly psychotherapy can be difficult, it is possible to use brief treatments and psychotherapeutically informed interventions. One major barrier is engagement: building trust with clients who may have experienced repeated failures or rejections in the healthcare system takes time and consistency, both of which are difficult to achieve when individuals are transient or mistrustful. Many homeless people prioritize basic needs such as food, shelter, and safety over mental health treatment, making psychotherapy seem like a distant concern. Additionally, it can be difficult to find a space where it is possible to have private conversations while traditional psychotherapy settings can be intimidating or inaccessible for individuals who are not housed. However systematic reviews of psychotherapy in people who are homeless have found that psychological interventions, particularly cognitive behavior therapy and motivational interviewing, can be effective for a range of outcomes [1].

10.1 Motivational Interviewing

Motivational Interviewing was developed by Miller and Rollnick [2] as a method to address ambivalence toward change, particularly in the context of substance abuse. It aims to create dissonance between what people do and what they say so that people will be motivated to change. For example, someone who says they want to be a good parent of young children but continues to overdose on substances is not consistent. The discomfort around dissonance aims to drive change. The core techniques include open-ended questions, affirmations, reflective listening, and

S. Hatcher et al., *Street Mental Health Handbook*,
https://doi.org/10.1007/978-3-032-00663-9_10

summarizing, often referred to by the acronym OARS. Motivational interviewing aims to elicit and strengthen "change talk"—client statements that favor change—while minimizing "sustain talk," or resistance to change [3].

Several studies have explored the effectiveness of motivational interviewing among people experiencing homelessness, particularly in addressing substance use, mental health issues, and engagement in services. A Campbell Collaboration systematic review of psychosocial interventions in people experiencing homelessness found evidence of a small effect of motivational interviewing on problematic substance use and mental ill health [4].

Substance Use Disorders Motivational interviewing has demonstrated some efficacy in reducing substance use among homeless individuals. A systematic review of motivational interviewing for reducing substance misuse in homeless populations found 11 randomized controlled trials [5]. The review concluded that motivational interviewing for substance misuse had a small but consistent advantage over usual care in adults especially for alcohol use.

Housing Retention and Health Outcomes The integration of motivational interviewing into housing-first models has also been associated with improved housing stability and health outcomes. In a trial by Gilmer et al. [6], motivational interviewing was incorporated into supportive housing interventions, resulting in better housing retention and lower rates of psychiatric hospitalization among participants.

Engagement with Primary Care O'Toole et al. [7] evaluated the use of a motivational intervention to improve engagement with primary care services among chronically homeless individuals. Their findings indicated that the motivational interviewing enhanced the likelihood of accessing primary care and improved continuity of care at 6 months (although the effect was markedly improved by also including an orientation visit to the clinic).

Despite promising evidence, the implementation of motivational interviewing in homeless services is not without challenges. Service providers often face high caseloads and limited resources, which can affect fidelity to motivational interviewing techniques. Additionally, staff may require extensive training and supervision to competently deliver motivational interviewing, particularly in complex cases involving cooccurring disorders. The transient nature of homelessness also means that sustaining long-term motivational interviewing interventions can be difficult, underscoring the importance of brief, opportunistic encounters. Cognitive impairment, which is common in the homeless population, can also make motivational interviewing challenging.

Combining motivational interviewing with harm reduction approaches, such as needle exchange programs and supervised consumption sites, aligns well with the stages of change model, meeting individuals "where they are" without imposing abstinence as a precondition for support.

10.2 Meaning and Logotherapy

For many of our clients it is difficult to find meaning in their lives. Sometimes the only meaning they will have is searching for and using drugs. Finding meaning is particularly important when people transition into housing and achieving basic safety needs are met. A particular form of therapy that focuses on meaning is logotherapy based on the writings of Viktor Frankl who survived the concentration camps of the holocaust in World War 2. He hypothesized that those who survived better in the camps were people who could maintain a sense of purpose or meaning—for him it was imagining himself giving a lecture on how people had survived in the camps (sic). Logotherapy helps people to find meaning through creative, experiential, and attitudinal values. Creative meaning comes from what people produce, create, and achieve often through work. Experiential meaning is acquired through experiences both positive and negative with other people including relationships, love, compassion, and shared moments. Attitudinal meaning comes from being true to your values such as taking a stand even when there are negative consequences. A Korean trial of eight sessions of logotherapy with homeless men, delivered by community mental health nurses, found significantly increased hope, empowerment, and meaning in life up to 4 weeks after the end of therapy [8].

Achieving meaning doesn't mean having to participate in therapy. In Ottawa, one of our programs implements a "block leader" role near a supervised injection site. These block leaders are recruited from the shelter population and receive compensation for their work. They wear high-visibility jackets identifying their role and patrol the area surrounding the site. Their responsibilities include maintaining cleanliness, collecting discarded drug paraphernalia, and assisting individuals who may be experiencing an overdose. Feedback from block leaders indicates that this role can be transformative, helping to restore self-esteem and bring meaning to their lives.

10.3 Trauma Therapy

Given the high prevalence of complex PTSD in the homeless population, trauma-focused therapy plays a crucial role. A scoping review [8] identified 28 studies specifically addressing PTSD and complex PTSD in vulnerably housed individuals. The review categorized interventions into four types: trauma-focused psychotherapies, non-trauma psychotherapies, housing interventions, and pharmacotherapies. Trauma-informed interventions were primarily small case series. Among the ten studies describing trauma-informed care, the most frequently cited elements were physical and emotional safety, the experience of feeling heard and understood, and flexibility of choice. Non-trauma focused therapies, including four randomized controlled trials, generally proved ineffective, which is consistent with the wider literature on treating PTSD. The literature also highlighted challenges in providing care to this population, such as, lack of private space for therapy delivery; cooccurrence of substance use; follow-up barriers, including limited length of stay in different shelters; and high staff turnover.

A trauma therapy designed explicitly for vulnerable populations is Narrative Exposure Therapy (NET), which is a short-term structured psychotherapy where the therapist helps the client reprocess traumatic memories so that they become more like normal memories and integrates them into a life story [9]. NET has been used with individuals who have experienced trauma including refugees, asylum seekers, street children, and survivors of organized violence. There is good evidence that NET can be effective in reducing PTSD symptoms and it can be especially useful in people who have experienced multiple traumas [10]. It can also be delivered by trained peers in settings where there are limited mental health resources.

There is some uncertainty whether it is beneficial to have a phased approach to starting trauma therapies. A phased approach involves a stabilization period of psychoeducation and skills training prior to confronting and processing past traumas. The period of stabilization is used mainly out of concern that confronting past traumas will overwhelm the client and lead to unhelpful coping strategies such as exacerbation of substance use. On the other hand, there is an argument that insisting on a period of stabilization restricts access to effective treatment for vulnerable groups and that there is little evidence that a period of stabilization results in better outcomes. In our experience of using NET with people who are homeless a period of education and engagement prior to starting therapy can be helpful to get people ready for therapy [11]. Even on its own educating people about complex PTSD and the effects of trauma on brains could be an intervention and a program specifically directed at people who are homeless would be useful. A systematic review of stabilization and phase orientated psychological treatment for PTSD concluded that stabilization interventions are helpful for reducing trauma symptoms and in preparing for trauma-focused therapy [12]. However, there was considerable variation in what counted as stabilization and none of the studies in the review was in a homeless population.

10.4 Cognitive Behaviour Therapy Including Problem Solving and Goal Setting

Helping people set goals and problem solving are important tools that all clinicians should have. Problem solving therapy is a way of teaching people a cognitive skill and giving them permission to stop and think [13]. The steps of problem solving involve recognizing when you have a problem by paying attention to feelings, thoughts, behavior, and somatic symptoms; brainstorming and choosing potential solutions; setting SMART goals; and then reviewing what happened to see if any changes are needed. SMART goals are Specific, Measurable, Achievable, Relevant, and Time Limited. For example, if a goal is to lose weight "I need to lose weight" is not a SMART goal. However, "I need to lose 2 kg in the next four weeks" is specific (2 kg), measurable (weight can be measured), achievable (it is feasible to lose 2 kg in 4 weeks), relevant (if chosen by the patient as an important goal), and time limited (4 weeks).

10.5 Contingency Management

Contingency management interventions aim to modify behavior by offering rewards, such as money, housing, or employment, for desired outcomes like negative urine tests. These interventions have primarily targeted substance abstinence, particularly from stimulants and alcohol, in homeless populations. A systematic review of contingency management for stimulant use revealed consistent improvements in outcomes, although the effect size varied considerably. Ethical concerns arise in these studies, particularly when linking negative urine tests to essential needs like housing or employment. A scoping review of financial incentives for behavior change in homeless populations found that 26 out of 29 studies reported significantly better outcomes for individuals receiving financial incentives compared to control groups [14]. However, contingency management's effectiveness is generally limited to individuals seeking substance abstinence. Several questions remain unanswered regarding the optimal frequency of rewards, the duration of interventions, and whether incentives should increase or decrease over time.

10.6 Housing First

The Housing First approach is based on the idea that housing should not be contingent on adherence to mental health treatment or substance abstinence. Instead, it considers housing a fundamental human right, to be provided regardless of an individual's mental health status or substance use. This model integrates housing provision with support services, often through case management delivered by Assertive Community Treatment (ACT) teams or similar.

A systematic review examining the efficacy of permanent supportive housing and income assistance for homeless individuals found that while Housing First interventions improved housing stability over 6 years, they did not significantly improve psychiatric symptom severity, substance use, or employment outcomes compared to usual care [14]. Notably, most studies in this review predated the North American opioid epidemic.

The lack of the effect on mental health and substance use suggests that different types of support than those based on assertive community treatment models are needed. Assertive treatment models primarily focus on people diagnosed with schizophrenia and use a model of shared care between team members. A model of care that is more trauma-informed and addresses the range of health issues common in people who have been homeless may be more effective in improving mental health outcomes.

10.7 Improving Discharge from Hospital

People experiencing homelessness spend a lot of time in hospital. They use hospital emergency departments five times more frequently than those who are housed, are admitted to hospitals three times as often, and have hospital stays three times longer

[14]. A cohort study comparing matched homeless and housed hospital inpatients showed that, after adjusting for health status on admission, homeless patients had 2.5 times the rate of emergency admissions, 0.6 times the rate of planned admissions, and 2.6 times the rate of ED visits compared to housed patients [15]. Once admitted, discharges are often characterized by being "against medical advice" or an unexpectedly prolonged admission. Additionally, people experiencing homelessness may be reluctant to stay in hospitals due to past traumatic experiences, fear of losing benefits or possessions, or concerns about withdrawal symptoms. Further, discharging people from hospital directly back to the streets or homeless shelters is seen as poor practice but inevitable given the lack of alternatives.

Discharging people experiencing homelessness has been described as a wicked policy issue characterized by complexity, a need to simultaneously focus on individuals and systems as well as integration across medical and social support organizations and professions [16]. Transitional care, which coordinates health and social support prior to hospital discharge, is based on critical time intervention theory, which aims to mobilize support during transitional periods [17]. In the UK, "Pathway teams" have been developed to assist homeless individuals being discharged from hospitals [18].

Evidence from randomized controlled trials suggests that transitional care schemes improve quality of life, reduce hospitalizations, and are cost-effective or cost-neutral. A 2022 systematic review of hospital-based transitional interventions for people experiencing homelessness found weak to moderate evidence for potential benefits in psychosocial outcomes, housing, healthcare use, and healthcare costs [19]. A realist review of the intermediate care literature focusing on hospital discharge of people who are homeless identified that the important components of intermediate care were consulting with service users, working in ways which are enabling, ensuring interprofessional collaboration and maintaining continuity of care [20]. Practical applications of these principles include involving service users in decisions about the timing and place of discharge; recognizing engagement with service users as a distinct clinical skill that needs to take into account past trauma; directly addressing stigma and discrimination; and providing physical rehabilitation and outpatient services tailored to the needs of homeless individuals.

10.8 The Importance of Good Endings

Many people we see who are homeless will have a history of bad endings for example being suddenly removed or put into care, sudden deaths in their social network or relationships marked by sudden absences. The consequence of this is that people will often try to avoid endings by provoking termination or withdrawing so at least they will have some control over the consequences. However, endings are unavoidable and as clinicians one of the things we can do is give people "the gift of a good ending." Good endings mean resisting the urge to ghost, or to cut off without explanation, or to leave things unsaid. Instead, it's a choice to honor the connection for what it was, to acknowledge the shared moments, and to part with respect. This kind of ending does not erase pain, but it can transform it, making space for growth rather than resentment. A good ending is an integral part of trauma-informed care.

Good endings are marked firstly by recognizing and naming endings. For example, letting someone know when their worker is going to leave or acknowledging the death of someone. Next reviewing what happened during the time of the relationship, what changed, what went well and what didn't go so well. Lastly by talking about the future what is going to happen next, lessons learnt, what goals are important and what is going to be different. It is also important to mark endings by rituals whether this is a funeral or memorial for someone who has died or a card or small gesture acknowledging the ending. Giving the gift of a good ending requires courage and presence. It asks us to face discomfort, to resist avoidance, and to engage fully with endings rather than rushing past them. A good ending is a recognition of value, of shared time, and of the fact that how we end things often matters as much as how we begin. To paraphrase a popular quote "endings define our lives – they are the fence posts on which the rest of our lives hang."

References

1. Bodley-Scott E, Ward RJ, Tarabay J, Fagbamigbe AF, Barker S, Maguire N. The effectiveness of psychological interventions for people experiencing homelessness: a systematic review and meta-analysis. J Community Appl Soc Psychol. 2024;34(5). https://doi.org/10.1002/casp.2863.
2. Miller WR, Rollnick S. Motivational interviewing: preparing people to change addictive behavior. [Internet]. J Commun Appl Soc Psychol. New York: Guilford Press; 1991 [cited 2025 Apr 26]. Available from: https://onlinelibrary.wiley.com/doi/full/10.1002/casp.2450020410.
3. Miller WR, Rollnick S. Motivational interviewing helping people change [Internet]. The Guilford Press; 2023 [cited 2025 Apr 26]. Available from: https://www.guilford.com/books/Motivational-Interviewing/Miller-Rollnick/9781462552795?srsltid=AfmBOoosZt1ix8vrJi_an4tQyhfd84RyHovfnliH2hpEj5jB55qW8DOB.
4. O'Leary C, Ralphs R, Stevenson J, Smith A, Harrison J, Kiss Z, et al. The effectiveness of abstinence-based and harm reduction-based interventions in reducing problematic substance use in adults who are experiencing homelessness in high income countries: a systematic review and meta-analysis: a systematic review. Campbell Syst Rev [Internet]. 2024 [cited 2025 Feb 2];20(2). Available from: https://pubmed.ncbi.nlm.nih.gov/38645303/.
5. Orciari EA, Perman-Howe PR, Foxcroft DR. Motivational Interviewing-based interventions for reducing substance misuse and increasing treatment engagement, retention, and completion in the homeless populations of high-income countries: an equity-focused systematic review and narrative synthesis. Int J Drug Policy. 2022;100:103524.
6. Gilmer TP, Stefancic A, Ettner SL, Manning WG, Tsemberis S. Effect of full-service partnerships on homelessness, use and costs of mental health services, and quality of life among adults with serious mental illness. Arch Gen Psychiatry [Internet]. 2010 [cited 2025 Apr 25];67(6):645–52. Available from: https://jamanetwork.com/journals/jamapsychiatry/fullarticle/210805.
7. O'Toole TP, Johnson EE, Borgia ML, Rose J. Tailoring outreach efforts to increase primary care use among homeless veterans: results of a randomized controlled trial. J Gen Intern Med [Internet]. 2015 [cited 2025 Apr 25];30(7):886–98. Available from: https://link-springer-com.proxy.bib.uottawa.ca/article/10.1007/s11606-015-3193-x.
8. Hyun M, Kim S, Park E. Effect of a logotherapy-based empowerment program for achieving self-reliance among persons living houseless. 2024 [cited 2024 Dec 22]. Available from: https://doi.org/10.1080/01612840.2024.2404691.

9. Narrative Exposure Therapy Institute [Internet]. [cited 2025 Apr 27]. Available from: https://www.net-institute.org/whatisnet.
10. Lely JCG, Smid GE, Jongedijk RA, Knipscheer JW, Kleber RJ. The effectiveness of narrative exposure therapy: a review, meta-analysis and meta-regression analysis. Eur J Psychotraumatol [Internet]. 2019 [cited 2025 Apr 27];10(1):1550344. Available from: https://pmc.ncbi.nlm.nih.gov/articles/PMC6450467/.
11. Edgar NE, Bennett A, Dunn NS, MacLean SE, Hatcher S. Feasibility and acceptability of Narrative Exposure Therapy to treat individuals with PTSD who are homeless or vulnerably housed: a pilot randomized controlled trial. Pilot Feasibility Stud [Internet]. 2022 [cited 2025 Apr 27];8(1). Available from: https://pubmed.ncbi.nlm.nih.gov/35428344/.
12. Willis DN, Dowling APC, O'Reilly PG. Stabilisation and phase-orientated psychological treatment for posttraumatic stress disorder: a systematic review and meta-analysis. Eur J Trauma Dissoc. 2023;7(1):100311.
13. Nezu AM, Nezu CM, D'Zurilla TJ. Problem-solving therapy: a treatment manual. New York: Springer Publishing Company; 2012.
14. Office of the Chief Analyst D. Healthcare for Single Homeless People Office of the Chief Analyst [Internet]. 2010 [cited 2023 Jul 9]. Available from: https://www.housinglin.org.uk/_assets/Resources/Housing/Support_materials/Other_reports_and_guidance/Healthcare_for_single_homeless_people.pdf.
15. Lewer D, Menezes D, Cornes M, Blackburn RM, Byng R, Clark M, et al. Hospital readmission among people experiencing homelessness in England: a cohort study of 2772 matched homeless and housed inpatients. J Epidemiol Community Health (1978). 2021;75(7):681–8.
16. Albanese F, Hurcombe R, Mathie H. Towards an integrated approach to homeless hospital discharge: an evaluation of different typologies across England. J Integr Care. 2016;24(1):4–14.
17. Critical Time Intervention | CTI Model | Critical Time Intervention.
18. Hewett N, Buchman P, Musariri J, Sargeant C, Johnson P, Abeysekera K, et al. Randomised controlled trial of GP-led in-hospital management of homeless people ('Pathway'). Clin Med [Internet]. 2016 [cited 2025 May 3];16(3):223. Available from: https://pmc.ncbi.nlm.nih.gov/articles/PMC5922699/.
19. Luchenski SA, Dawes J, Aldridge RW, Stevenson F, Tariq S, Hewett N, et al. Hospital-based preventative interventions for people experiencing homelessness in high-income countries: a systematic review. EClinicalMedicine. 2022;54:101657.
20. Cornes M, Whiteford M, Manthorpe J, Neale J, Byng R, Hewett N, et al. Improving hospital discharge arrangements for people who are homeless: a realist synthesis of the intermediate care literature. Health Soc Care Community [Internet]. 2018;26(3). Available from: https://www.ncbi.nlm.nih.gov/pubmed/28730744.

Index

S. Hatcher et al., *Street Mental Health Handbook*,
https://doi.org/10.1007/978-3-032-00663-9

MIX
Papier aus verantwortungsvollen Quellen
Paper from responsible sources
FSC® C105338

If you have any concerns about our products,
you can contact us on
ProductSafety@springernature.com

In case Publisher is established outside the EU,
the EU authorized representative is:
Springer Nature Customer Service Center GmbH
Europaplatz 3, 69115 Heidelberg, Germany

Printed by Libri Plureos GmbH
in Hamburg, Germany